"It is said there is a miracle medicine food for every organ that cures specific ailments. Here are MIRACLE MEDICINE FOODS... that have relieved or cured almost every known ailment—even when drugs and surgery failed!" says Rex Adams.

"So safe that no prescription is needed, so powerful that certain medications have had to be eliminated," Adams reports that "now—after years of research—their stories can be told."

"I find myself wanting to tell them all at once," he exclaims. And in this book, he brings the results of 15 years of work in writing and researching in the field of natural and drugless medicine and his own miraculous cure from a nearly fatal ailment together for you to consider.

MIRACLE MEDICINE FOODS

ABOUT THE AUTHOR

REX ADAMS began his brilliant career as a Medical Research Reporter, after graduating with highest honors from an Eastern preparatory school and the City University of New York. His genius having been recognized early, he was appointed Secretary to the President of a New York Medical Association at the age of 19. At 21, he became Administrative Assistant to the head of a major New York publishing company. At 23, he headed his own literary agency. At 24, he was Executive Vice President of another publishing company. For nearly 15 years, he has been writing and researching in the field of natural and drugless medicine.

ATTENTION: SCHOOLS AND CORPORATIONS

WARNER books are available at quantity discounts with bulk purchase for educational, business, or sales promotional use. For information, please write to: SPECIAL SALES DEPARTMENT, WARNER BOOKS, 666 FIFTH AVENUE, NEW YORK, N.Y. 10103.

**ARE THERE WARNER BOOKS
YOU WANT BUT CANNOT FIND IN YOUR LOCAL STORES?**

You can get any WARNER BOOKS title in print. Simply send title and retail price, plus 50¢ per order and 50¢ per copy to cover mailing and handling costs for each book desired. New York State and California residents add applicable sales tax. Enclose check or money order only, no cash please, to: WARNER BOOKS, P.O. BOX 690, NEW YORK, N.Y. 10019.

Miracle Medicine Foods

REX ADAMS

WARNER BOOKS

A Warner Communications Company

WARNER BOOKS EDITION

Copyright © 1977 by Parker Publishing Company, Inc.
All rights reserved.

This Warner Books Edition is published by arrangement with
Prentice-Hall, Inc., Englewood Cliffs, N.J. and Parker Publishing
Company, Inc., West Nyack, New York

Cover design by Tony Greco

Warner Books, Inc.,
666 Fifth Avenue,
New York, N.Y. 10103

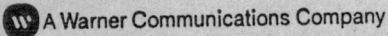 A Warner Communications Company

Printed in the United States of America

First Warner Books Printing: May, 1981

10 9 8 7 6 5

Contents

1. Miracle Medicine Foods For Instant Pain Relief! — 9
2. Miracle Medicine Foods For Bronchitis, Asthma, Emphysema and Lung Problems! — 29
3. Miracle Medicine Foods For Heart, Veins, and High Blood Pressure! — 47
4. Miracle Medicine Foods For Liver and Gall Bladder Problems! — 71
5. Miracle Medicine Foods For Kidney, Bladder, and Urinary Problems! — 83
6. Miracle Medicine Foods For Diabetics! — 97
7. Miracle Medicine Foods For The Stomach! — 107
8. Miracle Medicine Foods For Constipation, Diarrhea, Colitis, and Other Intestinal Ailments! — 119
9. Miracle Medicine Foods For Eyes, Ears, Nose and Throat! — 133
10. Miracle Medicine Foods For Hay Fever and Allergies! — 153

11	Miracle Medicine Foods For The Nerves!	165
12	Miracle Medicine Foods For Women's Problems!	187
13	Miracle Medicine Foods For Men's Problems!	209
14	Miracle Medicine Foods For The Skin!	225
15	Miracle Medicine Foods For Arthritis!	247
16	Miracle Medicine Foods For New Youth!	277

Miracle Medicine Foods

1

Miracle Medicine Foods For Instant Pain Relief!

When you hurt, you want quick pain relief, and there are miracle medicine foods—common foods, available everywhere —that can bring instant and immediate relief from the most horrible pains imaginable. In minutes, and even seconds, these foods have relieved great agony, avoided surgery, and cured the incurable in so many cases, I find myself wanting to tell them all at once!

Miracle medicine foods, available without prescription, that may instantly relieve the unimaginable torment of ulcers, arthritis, kidney and gallstones, urinary problems, relieve heart, lung and artery pains at once!

Instant pain relief for scores of ailments, and spectacular cures are reported with these miracle medicine foods from your garden, corner grocery, or health food store. In fact, many of these foods contain actual ingredients from which pain-relieving miracle medicines are made. While not a substitute for qualified medical care—always obtain your doctor's permission before using—these foods are reportedly safe and harmless, and can miraculously speed up the healing process so that ailments vanish in an amazingly short time!

Reported Cases:
- **You'll see how a man who was horribly scalded from head to foot by boiling water received immediate, in-**

stant, and complete relief—and escaped completely unharmed—with a miracle medicine food!
- An elderly woman was admitted to a hospital with gangrene of the foot, but after examining her the doctors decided she could not survive an amputation. It was decided to try this same amazing food. Her foot was actually tied in a bag full of it. To everyone's amazement, the foot soon healed, and she walked away completely cured!
- An 83-year old man with knee pain so bad "I could barely get up and answer the phone" discovered another miracle medicine food. He says: "Today I can keep stride with my younger friends, kick, jump or run without any discomfort whatever."
- A 53-year-old man with advanced spinal arthritis, tried another miracle medicine food you'll discover, and says: "In three days I could jump out of bed without dragging myself.... No more pain any more!"
- A man with a slipped disc, told by doctors he'd never get any better—and might even get worse—had suffered for 20 years in excruciating agony. Then he discovered a miracle medicine food. The first time he tried it, his disc slipped back into place, and he has been pain-free for 5 years!
- A woman with sharp leg pains tried a remedy you'll discover, and says: "Oh, what a comforting relief it was! Immediately, I felt a wonderfully refreshing feeling coursing through my legs... 10 minutes later, the pains were completely gone and (my legs) felt so strong and new! It was really amazing. The next day, the pain was still gone."
- A diabetic says: "I had to retire because I felt so weak. Doctors said there was no cure." Of the miracle medicine foods he'd discovered, he says: "I began this diet around 1920 and a year later the doctors could not find a trace of sugar. Now, at 70, I can eat anything on the table, and do more work than any man my age!"
- A man suffered angina (heart) attacks, and was told by doctors he had only 10 years to live, provided he avoid all exercise. He tried a miracle medicine food.

Twenty-two years later, he reported he has never had angina since!

- A 72-year-old woman with rheumatic heart, endocarditis, hardening of the arteries, and angina, says: "I had gotten to the place where I staggered when I first got out of bed or out of a chair." Then she discovered miracle medicine foods. Four weeks later, her EKG was normal!
- A man with varicose leg ulcers followed a doctor's advice for two years (ointments and ace bandages)— and was no better than the day he started. Then he discovered a miracle medicine food. In six weeks he had not one ulcer on his legs. They were completely healed!
- In one reported case, two gallstones were placed in a glass of tea containing a miracle medicine food. The next day, the stones were in four pieces. In five days they were like gravel. In 10 days they were completely dissolved!
- A man had x-rays showing gallstones. Friends told him about a miracle medicine food. Four days later, the gallstones passed. X-rays showed they were completely gone!
- A woman was having a gall bladder attack, with stabbing pains, nausea, and other symptoms. Touching a miracle medicine food to her side in a wet pack relieved her pains immediately, so strongly penetrating are its powers!
- A doctor wrote: "Fifteen years ago I was afflicted with the liver complaint. I used all my skill trying to cure it, but failed." Then he discovered a miracle medicine food, and said, "In almost every instance I have succeeded in restoring those who used this plant," including himself!
- A man suffering horrible kidney stones, with violent pains that tormented him constantly for 9 years—discovered a miracle medicine food. "I did not have to wait long for results," he says. "Large masses of uric acid crystals ... were excreted ... I was soon entirely free from my very great sufferings and have not had any trouble since."

- A woman with a swollen urethra had been to many doctors. They cut and treated and nothing helped. Then she tried a miracle medicine food, and says: "I've never had such results. It took out the swelling all over..."
- A man whose x-rays showed he had two ulcers, heard about a miracle medicine food for ulcers. He tried it and says: "Almost at once, there was no pain.... Both ulcers were healed when I had my checkup..."
- A man, suffering from a serious brain tumor and a stomach ulcer, with headaches and painful indigestion, was told by his doctor to try miracle medicine foods. In a short time, X-rays showed the ulcer vanished! Even more amazing, the brain tumor disappeared, and he was completely normal!
- Mr. D.R. reports: "My eyesight was so weak I could not read a printed page. Even large letters were blurry.... Soon I was wearing thick lenses." Then he discovered a miracle medicine food, and says: "In 2 weeks my vision cleared up. My doctor only shrugged and smiled. Why didn't he tell me this?"
- An elderly woman was told she had cataracts, and would need an operation. Instead, she used miracle medicine foods. Now she can see the numbers on a deck of cards, and has no more watery eyes.
- A woman with glaucoma reports the pressure in one eye was 36, and 32 in the other eye. She tried drops which did not lower the pressure, and irritated her eyes. Then she tried a miracle medicine food, and says: "Last week my pressures were taken and they were *normal*. My eye doctor couldn't believe it... he is going to tell his other glaucoma patients."
- A woman had heard nothing for 30 years, with her right ear, and very little with her left ear. Doctors had tried everything without success. Then she tried a miracle medicine food. and in a short time could hear a whisper!
- An elderly woman who'd been deaf for 20 years, tried a miracle medicine food, and was amazed to find she could hear without her hearing aid! She can hardly believe it!

- A lung victim was put on the operating table, where doctors found disease so widely spread they sewed him up and declared his case hopeless. Then he heard about a miracle medicine food and immediately started taking it. In 4 months, x-rays showed no sign of disease. He is back at his regular business!

To repeat, no one can guarantee instant pain relief or cures, nor is any food a cure-all for every ailment, but these foods to seem to have worked miracles in many reported cases, quickly relieving pain and suffering, and if just one of these foods can do this for you, or a loved one, it is truly a godsend!

Instant Pain Relief For Scores of Ailments!

In many cases, there are people who could not hobble around without drugs and constant agony, who now live totally pain-free, active, drug-free lives since using some of these miracle medicine foods.

Without drugs or surgery, heart attack and stroke victims —some barely able to walk—can now run! Clogged arteries opened up with increased blood flow and dramatic improvement! "It's a revolutionary breakthrough!" says one doctor of Miracle Medicine Foods. "Millions of lives can be saved!" Cholesterol can be reduced to nearly zero!

Lung and arthritis victims—ready for surgery—have been transformed from living skeletons barely able to shuffle a few feet, to hearty robust men and women who can run, kick, jump and keep stride with anybody. Now, after years of research, their stories can be told. And in my function as a medical research reporter, I'd like to tell you about them...

- The blind man whose sight was restored!
- Dying lung victims complete cured!
- Arthritic cripples who were completely healed!
- Gall bladder attack relieved in seconds!

- The failing heart that was rejuvenated!
- The bleeding hemorrhoids that vanished!
- The varicose veins that disappeared!
- Painful swollen limbs completely healed!
- How a man reduced 20 pounds in 12 days!
- The woman whose bladder infection healed!
- Seemingly hopeless cases of ulcers, spastic colon, colitis, constipation, diarrhea, liver and kidney fatigue quickly relieved!
- Diabetics completely cured without drugs!
- Prostrate trouble completely relieved!
- Hearing loss suddenly cured!
- Colds, flu, allergies, stuffed sinus and sharp head pains gone in minutes!
- How loose teeth took root again!
- How victims of baldness, gray or thinning hair, wrinkles, age spots, warts, bedsores, eczema, senility, trembling and old age symptoms were rejuvenated!

There are literally dozens of miracle rejuvenation foods listed in this book, with complete details on how they were used to relieve or cure specific ailments. Reportedly, you can turn off pain from many ailments, just like flicking a switch! Pain will vanish in seconds! To use this book is simplicity itself. A glance at the Contents page will tell you instantly where to look for answers to your specific problem, each chapter covering a specific ailment or area of the body. Let me give you an amazing preview of just one of these foods!

The Miracle Rejuvenation Plant!

Scientists have discovered an amazing healing plant that seems to relieve everyone of the signs and symptoms we associate with aging! A common plant—available everywhere for pennies without prescription!

In minutes, and even seconds this miraculous healing plant has relieved the agonies of liver, gall bladder, digestive and arthritic upset, merely by holding it against the skin, so penetrating are its powers!

Merely inhaling its fragrance has relieved or cured serious lung ailments! Partaking of its juice has healed heart, vein, artery, circulatory and high blood pressure problems! It is the most powerful antibiotic known in the form of pure food, with actual penicillin power!

Miraculous healing power seems to exist in this plant, said to relieve pains immediately, make illness vanish, fight infection, rejuvenate, even grow new hair—yet available at your local grocery. Spectacular cures are reported.

So safe that no prescription is needed—so powerful that certain medications have had to be eliminated under a doctor's care—there are people who were once unable to walk half a block without terrible pain who can now run, dance, swim and climb mountains, since using it!

It Has No Rivals! God Made It Unique!

In one sensational cure, a 19-year-old girl who was born with a short withered arm, that was paralyzed and useless was treated with a mild form of this miracle rejuvenation plant in hand baths and soaks, and was miraculously cured! Doctors said it was impossible! To prove it to a skeptical witness—she held out her hand and pinched him several times! The story appeared in all the Paris newspapers!

Records show people living well beyond 100 where this plant is eaten. One researcher found 40% of men over 90 still able to thread a needle without glasses! Doctors obtained sperm from a 119-year-old man! Heart disease and cancer were virtually unknown!

Sight and Hearing Restored!

Dimness of vision, impairment of the field of vision, blackouts, inability to focus or see up close, have all been corrected with a substance this plant activates for rejuvenated nerve health. Nerve-caused hearing loss has also been corrected! Louis D. had these middle-ear complaints. When this plant was added to his food, his hearing returned to normal. His vision with glasses was actually better than before, clear and sharp!

Poor Man's Penicillin!

It is the most powerful natural antibiotic known in the form of pure food! Against its juice, cold, flu, and virus germs don't stand a chance! It cuts phlegm, fights infections, clears sinuses, bronchial tubes, and lungs. It kills the most horrible germs, even leprosy, gonorrhea, and gangrene, in 5 minutes flat! In lab tests, these germs were actually hurled to the side of a culture dish. Reportedly, one tiny milligram of this plant had the same power as 25 units of penicillin!

Lung Ailments Cured!

Lung patients—near death's door—suffering all manner of respiratory ailments (asthma, emphysema, and horrible lung abscesses, allergies and bronchitis), have revived and walked away completely cured, praising this miracle rejuvenation plant! One researcher reports 90% of such sufferers were quickly relieved or cured!

Asthma & Emphysema Cured!

N.M., father of 5, was dying of asthma. His last attack nearly killed him, and he was afraid to move for fear of another seizure. With this miracle rejuvenation plant, he was cured, and had no more seizures! Myron E. could hardly breathe due to emphysema, with fits of wheezing, dizziness and heart pain. With this plant, all symptoms vanished! A serious allergy sufferer says, "It's like a new religious experience!"

Bladder Infection Relieved!

Mrs. N.Q. suffered from cystitis (inflammation of the bladder often with pain or burning on urination). She tried this plant in a simple drink, and had immediate relief! Her doctor told her about a lung cancer patient who survived all expectations eating this plant, no cure claimed!

Dog's Breast Tumors Disappear!

A woman reports that her poodle had breast tumors a vet said were probably malignant. The dog was given the juice of this plant. In 3 weeks, tumors gone!

Prostate Relieved!

D.J. had an enlarged prostate, causing difficult urination, frequent urges with bursting pains, painful infections, back pain. This plant gave him immediate relief, and he could urinate freely!

High Blood Pressure Relief!

In hundreds of tests, this plant reduces blood pressure, regardless of age or condition, often permanently! One doctor noted vast improvement in only one hour! In one case an overweight middle-aged man discovered that his pressure dropped from 190/90 to a mere 130/75, without dieting! It seemed safer and better than any drug!

Cholesterol Is Melted Away!

A major breakthrough is that the juice of this plant dissolves the gooey sludge involved in hardening of the arteries, according to two doctors! They said this plant could rid one of the build-up of fatty deposits on artery walls and help prevent arteries from clogging! The juice of this plant reduced cholesterol in test subjects who ate ¼ lb. of butter below fasting level!

Heart Symptoms Relieved!

A "heart juice" in this plant seems to stimulate the heart like digitalis ... relieving chest pain, headaches, dizziness, shortness of breath, opening clogged blood vessels, preventing them from bursting, increasing circulation throughout the body, dissolving deadly blood clots, soothing inflamation. It activates a substance (gives you 10 times more), said to strengthen weak heart muscles and reduce an enlarged heart in 2 days, according to a Harvard doctor!

A Startling Fact About Diabetes!

In *Lancet,* the British medical journal of December 29, 1973, two doctors report that this miracle rejuvenation plant is as effective as a popular drug in clearing the blood of excess sugar! It reportedly normalizes low blood sugar as well!

In one reported case, a man with diabetes and high blood pressure was told by doctors his case was incurable, and was sent home to die, at age 60. At age ninety he was still alive, in excellent health! He started eating this plant! His blood sugar dropped 200+ to 110! He passed the secret along to others, and all reported the same amazing relief!

Blessed Relief From Arthritis!

A French researcher claims 90 percent effectiveness in treating arthritis with this miracle rejuvenation plant! No special diet need be followed, he states, and he finds the plant so penetrating he applies it directly to the skin, in special soaks. Painful attacks of rheumatism, neuralgia, sciatica (leg pain), and gout disappeared!

A Cripple Walks Again!

Whenever Pete M. tried to stand up, he felt excruciating pain in his hip and leg. It felt like the hip was dislocated, as painful as sharp nails. He couldn't put his weight on it or make it move normally. In his leg he felt the high whining pain of phlebitis. With this amazing plant, he was able to walk painlessly once again—and the attacks never returned!

Arthritic Fingers Freed of Pain!

Jerome S. couldn't even hold a pencil or dial a phone due to arthritic fingers that were gnarled, swollen and painful. Nothing helped. Drugs made him ill. He even tried cutting out his favorite foods. With this miracle rejuvenation plant, he found immediate relief. Swelling and pain vanished! He regained his iron grip!

Spine And Shoulders Relieved!

Jane A. developed painful arthritis at the base of her spine, that made it impossible to sit. She could no longer do housework or straighten up—she had to be pulled to a standing position. Then she developed agonizing bursitis of the shoulders and couldn't move. With the juice of this amazing plant her spine became free and flexible, pain vanished in her shoulders and she moved easily!

Soothes Stomach and Digestion!

This plant is reported 95 percent effective in healing digestive upset. It brought not just temporary but permanent relief, in many cases. It has an almost narcotic-like effect in soothing the system. It relieved cramps and spasms (colitis). It contains 529 milligrams of a laxative, which has relieved constipation minutes after it was taken. In cases of diarrhea, it has worked miracles in stopping even the extreme diarrhea of dysentery. Nearly 100 percent of ulcer patients were cured in experiments testing a substance it activates in large quantity—a bleeding ulcer was healed in minutes!

Senility, Trembling, Paralysis And Old Age Symptoms Reversed!

Among users, the most striking effect was on the skin of the face, throat, arms and hands: the skin became smooth, taut and young-looking, lines and age spots faded away! A man nearing 70 suffering senile loss of memory regained his quick, sharp mind! Another whose hands shook violently became steady and calm. A woman with heart symptoms and paralysis was given this plant to eat: her heart symptoms subsided, and in a short time she got up and walked!

Rejuvenates Male And Female Glands!

Described as a cure for impotence and an aphrodisiac beyond compare, when a substance in it was given to men who were short, and had the genitals of children, almost immediately their genitals grew to normal size, and they grew taller. In fact, one gained five inches in height! In women, the plant is used to relieve inflammation of the uterus and menstrual cramps! A mild form of this plant—used as a popular candy flavoring (licorice), contains the female hormone estrogen. A substance it gives in large quantity has completely relieved the almost constant nausea of pregnancy!

Amazing New Help For Skin and Hair!

Crow's feet, jowls, double-chin, puffy bags and dark circles under the eyes have all vanished with this miracle rejuvenation plant Reportedly, the juice of this plant has caused bald spots to fill in and new hair to grow in many cases. In every case the hair grew in thick, dark and luxurious, regardless of age or sex. Blisters ... bedsores ... warts ... shingles ... unbearable itching ... athlete's foot ... boils ... insect bites and more, have completely vanished, sometimes overnight or in only minutes!

How To Loose 20 Pounds In 12 Days!

This miracle rejuvenation plant seems to melt off pounds faster than anything else in the world! No calorie counting or willpower is needed! Recently a national newspaper told how a famous actor uses this plant to lose over a pound a day, or about 10 pounds a week! While making a movie, he used it to lose 20 pounds in 12 days! This method is completely safe, according to a consulting dietician! Thighs, hips, buttocks, neck—all the hard-to-reach areas—seem to slenderize. Even shoe size is reduced!

Nature's All-Purpose Miracle Remedy!

If ever there was a miracle, practically all-purpose remedy, you've got it—not in your medicine chest—but in your vegetable garden! Garlic, the little vegetable that gave immortal strength to those who built the pyramids! Garlic, the stamina food that powered warriors, gladiators, and Olympic athletes, and enabled Alexander's troops to withstand the extremes of mountain cold and desert heat, to conquer the world! Prized and cherished even today, as explosive news reports continue to reveal amazing facts about it!

Fights Germs Penicillin Won't Touch!

In 1948, after years of research, scientists firmly established garlic's "penicillin power," by isolating various substances in it.

Alliin, the first substance isolated, was effective against the germs that cause salmonella poisoning, dysentery, and the staphylococci germs that cause skin boils and running sores. It was also effective against the streptococci germs that cause scarlet fever, sepsis, diphtheria, erysipelas, inflammation of the lining of the heart (rheumatic fever). *Alicin*, the other garlic ingredient, fights conjunctivitis (eye infection), putrefaction (food decay in stomach and intestines), typhoid, cholera and TB. But the big point to remember is that garlic is able to combat some germs even penicillin won't touch, like baccillus paratyphoid-A, which creates confusing symptoms like dysentery, "fake influenza," rheumatism, or kidney complications. Garlic vapors halt germs at a distance of 20 cm! Its germ-killing power remains in the bloodstream for 10 hours!

> During World War II, thousands of tons of garlic were purchased by the British government for treating wounds. It had been reported that not one case of septic poisoning or gangrene occurred among those treated! Around this time Albert Schweitzer reportedly used it against typhus, cholera and leprosy. In Malmo, Sweden, during a polio epidemic, out of 1,204 children who took it, not a single case occured. A Japanese doctor reports its effect against gonorrhea!

The only warnings I have ever seen in print with regard to garlic are that it should be cooked—or diluted—for people with weak constitutions, avoided by those with an allergy to sulfur, and not placed directly on open wounds. The Russians used special containers filled with ground garlic placed directly over an infected wound—even in amputation cases. The vapors alone killed any germs, and soldiers' wounds were cleaned quickly and efficiently!

Renewal of Youth and Health!

Dr. M.W. McDuffie used garlic to cure practically hopeless TB cases brought in on stretchers and wheelchairs, expecting to die. In the *North American Journal of Homeopathy*, May 1914, he calls it "the best individual treatment found to get rid of germs," and says, "If garlic is not a universal remedy and a renewer of health and youth, it appears at least to come nearer to that dream than any known thing given by nature for the use of man. It is all quite simple and entirely natural."

More Spectacular Cases!

That's just *one* miracle food, out of many revealed in these pages. You can see why I want to give these secrets to the world! Results are amazingly fast, bringing relief often in a matter of seconds. They require no expense, no special equipment in most cases, and can be used by anyone in perfect safety. Here you'll find scores of actual letters from people telling of the automatic pain relief they are getting with these miracle medicine foods!

- **One woman with two large breast tumors was about to have surgery. In the meantime, her doctor told her to use a miracle medicine food for relief of pain. Pain was completely relieved, the nodes became so small, the doctor decided not to operate, and finally they disappeared!**
- **A woman with breast lumps discovered that as soon**

as she used a miracle medicine food, "the pain and swelling would go away immediately." Without this remedy, she says, "I don't know what I'd do."
- For 25 years, one man reports he suffered from hay fever. Then he discovered a miracle medicine food, and ate some. The hay fever vanished in seconds, and each time it recurred, the same simple remedy banished it!
- A woman suffered 16 years with allergies, asthma, and nasal polyps. Medication, shots, diet, inhalants, cardiograms, blood tests, hypoglycemia tests, oxygen masks, extra dental work and seven nose operations for the removal of 130 polyps still left her miserable and short $25,000! Then someone told her about a miracle medicine food. She says: "The results are worth shouting about. . . . I have come back from a gasping, wheezing individual with my nose grown shut . . . to one with endless enthusiasm and strength!"
- An 80-year-old woman suffered a vaginal condition known as leukoplakia. Her doctor treated her with hormones, salves, etc., and she became worse. A specialist said her system had dried out due to a hysterectomy 35 years ago, and he could do nothing. She was in so much misery with her raw, burning area, she could not sit, stand or walk. Then she discovered a miracle medicine food. In a few days she felt much better. In a month, her misery was completely gone!
- A woman with hemorrhoids so bad she could not sit or lie down, asked a friend for advice. "What she told me to do brought immediate relief and is absolutely amazing!" Using a miracle medicine food, she says: "Within 30 minutes I could feel the pain being drawn out. . . . I am not exaggerating when I tell you that . . . I felt great and slept through the entire night."
- A man with hemorrhoids says that, after suffering several years, he discovered a miracle medicine food. "The effect," he says, "was miraculous. Application was made once a day for 2-3 days and the enlarged hemorrhoids completely disappeared. They have not returned. This cure happened after everything else had failed."

- A woman says: "I used to be constipated all the time for years, getting relief only from enemas." She discovered miracle medicine foods, and says: "Now ... I have two or three bowel movements every day."
- Another says: "For 7 years I did not have a normal bowel movment ... I went to doctors, who made me worse with prescriptions. I felt I was a hopeless case until a friend told me about (a miracle medicine food). For 59 cents I got relief."
- A woman with diarrhea says: "I had (it) for a long time, and was so weak I could hardly move.... Every time I stopped taking the doctor's prescription, the diarrhea came back worse." Then she tried a miracle medicine food, and says, amazingly, her diarrhea ceased almost immediately!
- Another woman had menstrual cramps constantly, but ever since she discovered a miracle medicine food, she says, "I have hardly any. It's hard to believe, but it is the only thing I'm taking that I didn't take before."
- One woman suffered such painful, heavy periods that even aspirin did not relieve them. The bleeding was almost hemorrhagic. Then she tried a miracle medicine food, and in 20 minutes the pain was gone and the bleeding stopped!
- A man with swollen prostate had complete stoppage of urine. A doctor told him he needed surgery. Instead, he used a miracle medicine food. Afterwards, he could urinate freely, and has not had any trouble since!
- A man who was impotent felt humiliated by this condition, tried a miracle medicine food, and felt a sudden surge of power such as he had not felt in 20 years, and the embarrassing condition never returned!

Here Are Fully Documented Facts ...

Startling evidence, pro and con, some of it overwhelmingly convincing, is presented. As in most health-related matters, use of ordinary non-prescription foods as medicine is controversial. Some doctors praise them to the sky, use them themselves, and recommend them to all their friends. They are considered minority unorthodox practitioners. Others violently disagree and say that such things are totally worthless, or should not be used by lay practitioners.

... And A Word Of Advice!

It is not the purpose of this book to delay the timely services of a doctor. You are advised to seek a doctor's advice immediately—for any condition which has been bothering you. All recognized authorities state that self-medication is inadvisable, without a doctor's approval.

The author completely endorses this, emphasizing that there is no substitute for a doctor. No two patients are alike. No single program can satisfy everyone. That's why the directions in this book are not to be considered prescriptions for any ailment you may have, and no attempt should be made to use them without your doctor's okay. Since I am neither a physician, consultant, or medical practitioner, I have not undertaken and will not undertake to diagnose or prescribe for any disease.

I claim only that many of these miracle medicine foods have worked for others. No such claimed effectiveness can be made for anyone else. That is for you—the reader—to decide, with your doctor. This book is a reference work only, based on my research and experience. Use for any other than its stated purpose is clearly contrary to my intent. And it should not be construed as an endorsement of any commercial food product.

Blessed Relief and Freedom from Pain!

For the blind, the deaf, the weak, the paralyzed and all those afflicted with common and uncommon ailments that refuse to yield to conventional medical treatment—for those beset with crippling pain who yearn to lead normal pain-free lives once more ...

For those who seek an instant and immediate end to devilish long-standing health problems that have been plaguing them and playing havoc with their lives and pocketbooks, defying all known orthodox treatments...

For those whose doctors have shrugged in bewilderment, unwilling or unable to suggest any avenue of relief beyond pills, potions, and medieval torture therapies that have not worked, and often seem worse than the ailment itself...

For seemingly hopeless cases, now ready to try Miracle Medicine Foods that have worked for tens of thousands just like them, down through the ages—for those who have knocked on every door, seeking help to no avail... this book promises miraculous new hope!

Suddenly no more lung pain... no more heart attacks ... no more high blood pressure or varicose veins... no more liver problems, gall bladder attacks, or burning urine... no more headaches, fatigue, diabetes or low blood sugar... no more constipation, colitis, ulcers or burning hemorrhoids... no more joint inflammation or stiffness... no more spasms... no more foggy vision or poor hearing... no more hay fever, sinus headaches, or skin problems... in case after reported case!

When you hurt, you want the fastest, easiest, safest and most reliable and inexpensive relief you can get—the major problem being where and how? When time is short, and pain is overwhelming, you cannot wait for Medical Science to come up with a possible remedy in the distant future. This book is the where and how of fast, easy, inexpensive pain relief—based on the true-life experiences of others. It is said there is a Miracle Medicine Food for every organ that cures specific ailments. Here are miracle medicine foods that have relieved or cured almost every known ailment—even when drugs and surgery failed! Automatic pain-relieving foods so powerful they may be called Bionic Healing Foods!

Thousands report spectacular cures and instant pain relief for scores of ailments with Miracle Medicine Foods, said to relieve pains immediately, make illness vanish, kill germs, fight infection, with actual penicillin power! So safe no prescription is needed. So powerful certain medications have had to be eliminated under a doctor's care! They include food supplements, massage or anything else that helps sufferers. All are foods, for if they help in any way they are Miracle Medicine Foods for the body!

2

Miracle Medicine Foods For Bronchitis, Asthma, Emphysema And Lung Problems!

Honey is *miracle medicine food* for bronchitis, asthma and lung infections. It relieves inflammation and soothes painful coughing spasms. An ancient folklore remedy for bronchial complaints is to simmer 3-4 slices of onion and a couple of cloves of garlic in half a quart of Irish Moss jelly for 30 minutes. When cool, strain and add 4 ounces of honey. Take one teaspoonful every two hours, alternating with one teaspoonful of plain honey, sipped slowly, every hour!

Honey has a fatal effect on germs, which is mainly due to its moisture absorbing ability. Its power to do this is phenomenal. It can draw moisture from a stone or crock, or even from a metal or glass container! When germs come in contact with honey, all their moisture is withdrawn—they shrivel and die. It has killed the most harmful bacteria imaginable, with actual penicillin power!

The results are nothing short of spectacular! One man, Mr. J.F., reports that 40 years ago, he became ill and consulted several doctors, who said he had active tuberculosis. After a few months the doctors gave him up, and said his only hope was to go to Arizona, which he could not afford to do. Later, they told him flatly he had only a few weeks to live. He began using honey daily. Five years later, the same doctors examined him, and found only a few spots on his lungs. They absolutely refused to believe it was the same person.

Mrs. Lorna G. reports that as a young girl, she was given up by her physicians as a hopeless consumptive (TB). Someone prescribed a diet of honey and goat's milk, with the result that she was free of illness the rest of her life, and still spry and healthy at 90!

Vinegar Heals Serious Lung Infection!

A five-year-old girl developed a nagging cough, which exploded into a serious lung infection. Doctors gave her penicillin, streptomycin and aureomycin. She improved and then had a relapse. It was found that her problem was a germ—which no drug could touch—that was rampaging through her system because the antibiotics had killed away all its enemies. Other drugs were tried, without success.

Large cavities developed in both her lungs. It was impossible to operate because she was too weak. Then her doctor heard how diluted vinegar was used to treat 165 cases of ear infection, due to the same germ. He placed a vaporizer near her bed, containing 2 tablespoons of vinegar in a quart of boiling water, and had her inhale this for 15 minutes, three times a day.

The child improved and was able to go home. Treatments continued. She gained weight, her cough disappeared, and she is now living a normal life. In a medical article, the doctor states: "This inexpensive (vinegar vapor) method of treatment can be used in the home for patients with chronic pulmonary suppuration (lung infection with pus) for which surgical intervention is not suitable." Vinegar, a miracle medicine food that accomplished what penicillin could not!

30 Years of Suffering Ended Overnight!

A man reports that he suffered from asthma for 30 years. While standing by a fence, chatting with a neighbor, he absent-mindedly nibbled a bit of comfrey leaf. That evening, he seemed to feel better, and had his first night of restful sleep in years. He wracked his brain to remember what he had done that day to obtain such results. He reasoned it must be the comfrey leaf. Now he eats some every day and has not suffered from asthma since!

A Simple Tea Saves Thousands Of Dollars In Medical Bills!

Mr. C.Y., a serious asthma sufferer, states: "For years I have been under the care of various doctors for asthma. I have spent thousands of dollars on prescribed medication that at best gave but temporary relief.

"Then last summer, a friend of mine suggested that I try 8 ounces of mullein tea daily for my asthma. I did and for a time saw no results. Then slowly, I began to improve. Now I take no medication and feel wonderful. But I do drink mullein tea daily ...

"Mullein tea can be made from the green plant or the dried leaves and I enjoy it both hot or iced. I do not know that it will help anyone else like it did me, but it is free for the gathering. Too, it is delicious in flavor ... superior to regular tea."

Soya Oil Relieves The Incurable!

Intravenous infusions of soya oil have brought about more improvement in a small group of children with cystic fibrosis than any other treatment, according to Robert B. Elliott, M.D., a New Zealand physician (*Pediatrics,* April 1976).

Cystic fibrosis has no known cure. It attacks the victim's respiratory system with repeated infections, and also attacks the pancreas and large intestine. Children who are born with it rarely live more than a few years. With soya oil, however, Dr. Elliott was able to stop deterioration, and in one child it was actually reversed!

All seven children gained weight! In six, deterioration of the respiratory tract was halted! Soya oil was chosen because it contains linoleic acid, which victims apparently lack. Dosage by mouth proved ineffective. Compared with a group which did not receive soya oil, respiratory problems occurred much more frequently, lungs deteriorated considerably over the same period of time, and two died.

Cystic Fibrosis Victim Wins Second Place At Track Meet!

Dr. Elliott says, "the clinical progress of these reported cases appears to be more favorable than the best reported series so far. Concurrent with the weight gain is a feeling of 'well-being' resulting in such feats as that of an older boy ... who had previously been quite disabled and who came in second in his school track meet after eight months of Intralipid therapy."

Asparagus For Lung Victims!

A biochemist reports a number of cases in which asparagus seems to have cured the incurable: "One man had an almost hopeless case of Hodgkins disease, and he was completely incapacitated. Within one year from starting the asparagus therapy, his doctors were unable to detect any signs of (disease), and he is back on a schedule of strenuous activities."

Here is what he says about a lung victim: "On March 5, 1971, he was put on the operating table, where they found (disease) so widely spread that it was inoperable. The surgeons sewed him up and declared his case hopeless. On April 5 he heard about asparagus therapy and immediately started taking it. By August, x-ray pictures revealed that all signs ... had disappeared. He is back at his regular business routine."

This biochemist states: "Asparagus should be *cooked* before using, and therefore canned asparagus is just as good as fresh. ... Open the can and dump into a blender. Liquify at high speed to make a puree, and store in a refrigerator. Give ... 4 full tablespoons *twice daily*, morning and evening. Patients usually show improvements in from 2 to 4 weeks. It can be diluted with water and used as a cold or hot drink. ... Larger amounts can do no harm, and may be needed in some cases.... As a biochemist ... I believe ... asparagus used as we suggest, is a harmless substance. The FDA cannot prevent you from using it, and it may do much good."

Grape Juice for Weak Lungs!

In *Old-Fashioned Health Remedies That Work Best* (Parker Publishing Co., Inc., 1977), L.L. Schneider, D.C., N.D., says he recovered from pleurisy and a collapsed lung, using a grape juice diet to eliminate mucus and phlegm. He has remained on this diet as long as seven weeks, considers it miraculous, says nothing else has worked as well, and that it gives him amazing energy! In severe cases, he recommends that you eat nothing except undiluted, unsweetened grape juice, as much as desired, for three or four weeks (grapes may be eaten, as well). In less severe cases, he recommends a meat and grape juice diet (see Chapter 4). The grape juice seems to cleanse the blood of poisons. No cure, but amazing relief is claimed. He tells of a patient, Mrs. G., in her late sixties, with an advanced case of emphysema, and very labored breathing: 500 cc was all she could exhale. With this diet, in one week she was exhaling 2,000 cc, an improvement of three hundred percent! He reports another case of advanced emphysema, a mine worker, 63, who had a bloated belly due to labored breathing. He followed the diet faithfully, and his breathing improved rapidly—in fact, his bloated belly lost one inch per day, every day for a week!

Cranberries Bring Instant Relief for Asthmatic Wheezing and Lung Spasms!

One of Dr. Schneider's patients, a New England farmer, says that his grandmother used tasty red cranberries to stop his asthmatic wheezing. She would mash some through a strainer and add some warm water. A cup of this would cause an almost immediate opening of the bronchial tubes—just like adrenalin!

Answer To An Asthma Victim's Prayer!

Mrs. V.N. reports: "At the age of 4½ (my son) was struck with a serious attack of asthma, for no apparent reason, and it lasted a week. For two years after this, chronic attacks of asthma followed. We never knew when they would strike or how long they would last. Constant pediatric attention provided only temporary symptomatic relief with medication and vaporizers, and even with these cyanosis often appeared, and I believe that on several occasions it was only prayer that saved his life.

"We saw allergists, psychologists, specialists of every kind. We were advised to get rid of the dog, to have no wool around the house, to avoid feather pillows... but the pattern of acute, chronic asthma remained unchanged. Two Christmases in a row the child had pneumonia, and the second time I was nearly ready to collapse. At this time I went deep into prayer. I told God that I had tried and done everything I knew how to do for my son, and if there were to be an answer, it had to come from him.

"And something from reading came into my mind, that vitamin E increases the body's ability to utilize oxygen.... I figured there could be no harm in giving him 100 mg. daily of alpha tocopherol, and I started him, as he was convalescing from pneumonia (then age 6½) on this program.

"As of that day, eleven years ago, the attacks came to an end. We have had no more asthma, and no more pneumonia, even though we live in one of the most smog-congested areas of the country. Even though I have little control over the diet that a 17½-year-old boy consumes when he is at school or away from home, he rarely misses his supplements, which include (now) 200 units of vitamin E daily.

"I'm not saying vitamin E cures asthma! I'm saying that

my son who was in a fair way to become crippled with this disease over a period of two years, has had no further lung developments since the regular employment of alpha tocopherol in his daily diet." If vitamins, minerals or food supplements help in any way, they are clearly miracle medicine foods for the body.

Miracle Medicine Food For Instant Relief of Respiratory Ailments!

Nerve massage can be a miracle medicine food for your lungs. Reportedly rubbing the nerve ends on various parts of the body—which lead like telephone lines to the breathing system—can cause anesthesia, and blessed relief. Called Zone Therapy, Neuroflexation, Pointed Pressure Therapy or Acupressure, it may be used in the following manner, say experts:

> **For hay fever and asthma, massage the thumb of each hand until there are no more tender spots. Do the same for the next three fingers, including the webs between. Several time a day, keep steady pressure on the thumb, first and second finger for about 15 minutes by winding a rubber band around them, removing only to let the blood circulate.**

For emphysema and TB, massage all the fingers on both hands, with a press and roll motion, also pinching the webs, and the pads under the fingers. Use steady pressure to anesthetize or deaden pain, and a rotating motion to stimulate circulation to the lungs.

Reported Cases:
- One doctor reports that whooping cough can be cured simply and easily with this miracle medicine food. An ordinary case of whooping cough, which has persisted for weeks, can sometimes be cured in 3 to 5 minutes, he says—adding that it never fails to bring relief!
- Another doctor reports spectacular cures of asthma! He says that one woman had such bad attacks of bronchial asthma that she was living on drugs and could hardly

sleep, except for catnaps in a sitting position. With this miracle medicine food—in 5 minutes—for the first time in years, she was relieved of all pain and shortness of breath, and no longer needed any drugs!

- An elderly man had emphysema for years and could hardly breathe. After using this miracle medicine food for the lungs, he was able to take his first deep breath in 20 years! Instant relief!

Hopeless Victim Cured After Suffering 30 Years!

Maurice Mességué, in his book *Of Men and Plants*, records the case of Mr. Rameau, an engineer from Paris, who was suffering from chronic asthma. The man was physically exhausted. He had great difficulty breathing and had to pause every few seconds to catch his breath.

"Sir," he told the great French healer, "I have come to you because ... the doctors openly admit they can do nothing for me ... I have already consulted all the top men in the medical profession ...

"I've been a chronic asthmatic for over thirty years," he continued, "ever since I was gassed (in the war). My really bad attacks are so fierce that I've never been able to take up any employment, and when I'm not having an attack I'm in a state of suffocation. I have to sleep sitting bolt upright in a chair, and there are days when I can't even take a step up from the street to the sidewalk. It takes so much effort and courage and will power just to go on living that I've more than once thought of putting an end to it."

Mességué agreed to treat the man with his famous "macerations." Listed in the book is a remedy for asthma, the prime ingredient of which is garlic.

Three months after his first visit, Mr. Rameau declared: "Now I really dare believe I'm cured! ... My condition is so improved that I think I can go back to work!"[1]

---

[1] Reprinted with permission of Macmillan Publishing Co., Inc., from *Of Men and Plants* by Maurice Mességué. Copyright © 1972 by Weidenfeld & Nicholson Ltd. Copyright © 1973 by Macmillan Publishing Co., Inc.

An Age-Old Remedy For Breathing Problems!

Garlic is reportedly the oldest, safest, and surest remedy for asthma, bronchitis, and other respiratory ailments. For centuries, the Chinese, Greeks, and Egyptians all claimed that garlic cured infections of the respiratory tract. Dioscorides, a Greek physician who accompanied the Roman soldiers as their official doctor, in the 2nd century, specified garlic for all lung disorders. Pliny, the 1st century Roman naturalist, maintained that garlic cured consumption (TB). Down through the ages, garlic's reputation as an aid to breathing has persisted.

And this is because of garlic's proven antiseptic, germicidal powers. Grated garlic placed near the most vicious germs will kill them all in 5 minutes! Typhoid, cholera, polio, TB—even leprosy and gonorrhea—have all been stopped dead in their tracks by garlic! Against garlic, cold, flu, virus and allergy germs don't stand a chance!

In addition, the ethers of garlic are so potent and penetrating they dissolve mucus in the sinuses, bronchial tubes, and lungs. As one woman stated: "It was from an herb book that I learned about the wonders of garlic, and cleared up pneumonia congestion in my lungs when antibiotics failed." It is truly *Poor Man's Penicillin!*

Ninety Percent Relief Reported!

Among the best results that Mességué, the great French herbalist, has achieved are cases of asthma, bronchitis, and other respiratory ailments. Mességué, himself, does not care much for statistics. But one of Mességué's colleagues spent countless hours tabulating the results of Mességué's treatments. For respiratory ailments, the record shows[2]—

Ailment	Cured	Improved	Unknown
Asthma	60%	30%	10%
Bronchitis	10%	80%	10%
Emphysema	10%	70%	20%

[2] *Of Men and Plants* by Maurice Mességué, *Ibid.*

The cure—which involves garlic—was learned from Mességué's father, Camille. "He was successful in his treatment of asthma," states Mességué, "which in those days could be traced to simpler causes... Nowadays, air, water and food are polluted by chemicals which we then breathe or swallow. My father used to treat asthma with foot-baths. He would drop what he called his macerations into three or four liters of water, and his patients would soak their feet in this for quite a time."[3]

"Why the feet?" you ask. Why not? It doesn't really matter how you take garlic—its penetrative powers are so strong that even when applied to the soles of the feet its odor is exhaled by the lungs, within an hour!

Basic Preparations[4]

For allergies, asthma, bronchitis, and emphysema, Mességué uses garlic—in large doses—in combination with other herbs and spices, all available without prescription at most health stores and herbal pharmacies. These applications are for external use only (foot baths, hand soaks, hip compresses) and are not to be eaten, or taken internally. All of Mességué's treatments include the following basic preparations.

Dried roots should be crushed; semi-fresh roots should be grated. Fresh plants should be chopped. Garlic should be crushed. He warns the user to follow the exact dosages given, otherwise the plants give undesirable, and sometimes disagreeable effects.

For foot and hand-baths, boil two quarts of water and allowed to stand for five minutes. Add to this ½ pint of crushed or chopped plants and let "macerate" for four or five hours, protected from dust. Then pour into a clean bottle (never use a metal container, he says). The resultant prepara-

---

[3]*Mességué, Op. cit.*

[4]Reprinted with permission of Macmillan Publishing Co., from *Of Men and Plants* by Maurice Mességué Copyright © 1972 by Weidenfeld & Nicolson Ltd. Copyright © 1973 by Macmillan Publishing Co., Inc.

tion can be used for eight days, without boiling or adding more water.

ALLERGIES
Garlic (one crushed head)
Single seed hawthorn (blossom—one handful)
Greater celandine (flowers and stems, if possible semi-fresh—one handful)
Couch-grass (roots—one handful)
Common broom (flowers—one handful)
Sage (leaves—one handful)
Linden (blossom—one handful)

Use in foot and hand-baths.

ASTHMA
Garlic (one large crushed head)
Corn poppy (flowers and capsules—one handful)
Lavender (flowers—one handful)
Ground-ivy (leaves—one handful)
Parsley (leaves—one handful)
Sage (flowers—one handful)
Thyme (flowers—one handful)

Use in foot and hand baths. Mességué advises that since asthma stems from a variety of allergies, you should follow your doctor's advice. While this preparation can bring relief during an attack, it is not necessarily a cure.

BRONCHIAL DISEASES
Garlic (One large crushed head)
Borage (flowers and leaves—one handful)
Cabbage (fresh leaves—one handful) *or*
Corn poppy (flowers and capsules—one handful)
Watercress (fresh flowers—one bunch)
Sage (flowers—one handful)
Sweet violet (flowers—one handful)

Use in foot and hand baths. In cases of bronchial and pulmonary catarrh, the treatment is the same as above.

EMPHYSEMA
  Garlic (one large crushed head)
  Single seed hawthorn (blossom—one handful)
  Ground-ivy (leaves—one handful)
  Sage (flowers and leaves—one handful)
  Thyme (leaves—one handful)

Use in foot and hand baths.

* * *

Reported Results[5]

On a lecture tour in Morocco, Mességué was challenged by one of the doctors at a medical convention, and offered to treat an asthma patient deemed incurable. The patient was to accompany Mességué back to France—where he would be treated at Mességué's expense—and then returned to be examined by a panel of doctors.

The patient was a hairdresser, Narcose Murciano, father of five children, who was suffering from such severe chronic asthma that work had become impossible. His acute attacks were so serious that the last one had nearly killed him. His case was desperate.

The man was, in fact, so incredibly ill that Mességué thought he was dying. His skin had lost all its elasticity—it stuck together when pinched. "The journey to France was a nightmare." Mességué recalls. "The poor wretch had to be so careful not to waste any of what life he still had left that he made not the slightest movement. He even kept his eyes shut...."

Completely Cured!

"Two months later I took him back to Casablanca, completely cured," says Mességué, "and he has had no more attacks to this day.... Since then the doctors in Morocco have

---

[5] *Of Men and Plants* by Maurice Mességué, *Ibid.*

sent me every asthmatic who has failed to respond to traditional treatment."

Cured In Five Days!

In another case a Mr. Peyrot gave this testimony: "I had consulted more than twelve French and Swiss medical practitioners, all capable men, but none of them was able to relieve my attacks of asthma. I was suffocating day and night, and Maurice Mességué cured me in five days."

Doctor Admits Cure!

Dr. Kreps, a surgeon and professor at Basel University, states: "... it is my duty to tell you that this man (Mességué) cured my own wife, who had always suffered from chronic asthma, against which we were powerless."

How Garlic Works To Cut Phlegm, And Fight Infection!

Here is another testimonial. One of Mességué's patients, a Mr. Glenna, from the southern part of France, states: "I kept getting lung abscesses: as fast as one would heal, another would return.... The doctors had more than given me up. The last two doctors had told me there was no hope and my wife was already preparing to go into mourning when her sister, who lives in Nice, told her that Mr. Mességué was performing miracles with his plants. I believe in herbs, myself. He gave me poultices and foot-baths, and my doctor in Menton had to admit that I was cured."[6]

The Cure of Incurable Ailments!

Even positive thinking can be miracle medicine food for the lungs. In her book, *The Miracle of Metaphysical Healing* (Parker Publishing Co., 1975), Dr. Evelyn Monohan tells how this miraculous secret has worked for hundreds, and says

---

[6]*Of Men and Plants* by Maurice Mességué, *Ibid.*

it will bring a cure from all allergies, with a simple method she gives.

In fact, she says, this secret brings cures to diseases and injuries which many doctors consider virtually "incurable!" With this secret, she claims you have the power this very moment to experience a complete cure from any disease or injury, no matter how horrible its reputation, and quickly end all pain and suffering! It brings perfect health, she says.

That goes for many ailments associated with great pain, like ulcers, arthritis, heart ailments, and many more. She says you can experience absolute relief, often without medicines or surgery! In fact, she states flatly, this method is 100 percent effective in curing many ailments, when used faithfully.

It involves clearly visualizing the disease you wish cured, in a quiet place, relaxed, eyes closed, and visualizing it fading away, with positive affirmations that you will be cured—completely blotting out any negative thoughts, several times every day. You cannot fail with this technique, she says. "There is no physical disease, illness or injury that you cannot heal this way," she says, and as convincing proof she tells how many incurable ailments were cured, including her own blindness, paralysis, and epilepsy, 9 years of suffering, cured in 10 days!

Meditation Saves Dying Woman!

A variation of this is called "meditation therapy." The mind is made to dwell closely on what may best be described as a nonthought—nonsense words, like "dot . . . dot . . . dot." In meditation therapy, it's not that your thinking is different—it's that it practically ceases. The mind becomes like a hollow tube. And as the mind is "disconnected" from the body, the body heals, reportedly.

Mrs. Janis O., 45, was dying of disease that had spread to her stomach, spine and abdomen. She was in excruciating pain, unable to eat, and had lost 30 lbs. She had a bloated belly, her stomach and intestines had swelled,

over 10 pints of fluid were drained from her abdomen, and she had a lump in her groin. She was so exhausted from drugs, tests and expensive medical treatments, including a hysterectomy, and was so weak, she could barely climb the stairs to see her doctor.

Then she was given meditation treatments. Every day, in a quiet room, she was told to empty her mind of *all* thought by repeating meaningless words over and over. After 6 weeks of meditation, her doctor reports, strength began to return, her stomach and abdomen softened, the lump in her groin disappeared, and she could eat solid food again. Her pain vanished, and after nearly a year doctors say she is still improving, and quite active. For Janis O., meditation is clearly miracle medicine food, allowing the body to heal itself. (A doctor's supervision is required, no cure is claimed, and self-treatment is not recommended.)

Proof You Can be Healed Of All Diseases And Never Pay Another Doctor Bill!

Reginald D. MacNitt, Ph.D. gives many case histories "to prove that you can not only be healed from all diseases but that you can keep yourself well and free from all doctor bills for as long as you remain (on) earth," in his book *How to Use Astral Power* (Parker Publishing Company, Inc., 1977). "Some say they were cured instantly," or in a short time, he adds!

Reported Results:
- Dr. MacNitt says he almost died from a respiratory ailment. Astral Power saved his life, he says, and you can use this method to cure emphysema. He tells of a fireman, Duane L., who nearly lost his job due to "permanent" heart-lung damage. Astral Power repaired all the damage in little over a month, and saved him! It has cured psoriasis in 3 days, healed completely paralyzed legs in a week—stopped bleeding in 10 seconds!
- Helen had a uterine tumor about the size of a grapefruit

which was getting larger every day. The tumor was made up of dried blood that was not expelled during her monthly periods. She had undergone two operations during the past ten years for removal of this tumor. Now it was back again and she did not want a third operation. With this secret, Helen's tumor went away for good without surgery!

"There is no reason why anyone should spend vast sums of money buying pain killers, sleeping pills or chemical relaxers... your body will be healthy automatically and continually" with this secret, which can eliminate common aches and pains instantly, says Dr. MacNitt! Astral Power is a state of mind, he says. His formula for attaining it is Relax-Concentrate-Contemplate. Relaxing in a quiet room, undisturbed, you should learn to complete just six breathing cycles a minute, gradually diminishing to three a minute. During this time, he says, keep easing thoughts out of your mind, until you are completely unaware of your body. Then visualize what you want. Your mind will automatically begin a healing process. The final step is contemplating oneness with God and the Astral World—where the human spirit never dies, and where, in fact, you can commune with all great minds that ever lived. Ask for a healing. It can miraculously speed up the healing process, he says!

"Hundreds Will Be Cured and Save Thousands of Dollars!"

"Somewhere along the line, doctors made people believe they were dependent on them to keep the human machine going. Nothing could be further from the truth," says Dr. MacNitt. "Healing without drugs or surgery does exist and is an established fact." When more people discover this, he says, "hundreds will be cured and save thousands of dollars." When serious disease strikes, the doctor is often helpless, except through drugs or surgery, he says, adding: "Kick the doctor and drug habit." With this secret, he says, "A miracle a day keeps the doctor away." If Astral Power, Metaphysical Healing, Meditation therapy, or any other mind power method can do this, clearly, it is miracle medicine food! And it costs you nothing! It seems perfectly safe to use along with—not as a substitute for—qualified medical care.

3

Miracle Medicine Foods For Heart, Veins, And High Blood Pressure!

In his book, *The Low-Fat Way to Health and Longer Life*,[1] Lester M. Morrison, M.D. writes: "Now I'm going to tell you about one of the most important nutritional supplements developed in the last 50 years. Make a careful note of it and of how it is to be used, as described in these pages. The least it can do for you is to improve your health and give you added vitality. And it may help save your life." He goes on to describe soybean lecithin.

> Soybeans contain the miracle medicine food lecithin, an unsaturated fatty acid. Soybean lecithin has been found to clean out veins and arteries—dissolve the gooey sludge cholesterol—and thus increase circulation, relieve heart, vein and artery problems, soothe the liver and gallbladder (bile and gallstones contain cholesterol), relieve anemia, kidney disorders, eczema, psoriasis, and some forms of arthritis. It has cured many diabetics—cured brain clots, strokes, paralyzed legs, hands and arms!

Dr. Morrison says that lecithin is an essential constituent of all living cells and plays a vital role. After more than 10 years of intense experimentation, he says that lecithin is the

---

[1] Prentice-Hall, Inc., 1958.

best of all cholesterol-reducing agents tested, and can *prevent* heart and blood vessel disease. Atherosclerotic plaques are dissolved and removed by lecithin, he says, and soybean lecithin is able to prevent blood clotting in the arteries! In those who used it, scientists found evidence of increased immunity against virus infections (including immunity against pneumonia)! Dr. Morrison says he is certain that lecithin is one of our most powerful weapons against disease, and an especially valuable bulwark against development of hardening of the arteries and all the complications of heart, brain, and kidney that follow. He calls it the most valuable of all food oils!

Dr. Morrison places lecithin at the top of the list in a heart-food program of lean meats, soft fats (those that are liquid at room temperature, such as most vegetable oils), fish, poultry, fresh fruits and vegetables, all cooked or dry cereals, whole wheat bread, most natural syrups and honey, and fat-free beverages. He says to *include lecithin with certain powerful heart-food supplements at mealtime,* in a five-step program as follows: (1) take 2 to 4 tablespoons of soybean lecithin at breakfast, (2) add the most powerful dose of B complex vitamins you can get in tablet form (follow the instructions on the label but ask your dealer for the best brand), (3) take at least 25,000 units of vitamin A and 150 mg. of vitamin C daily, (4) take two tablespoons of soybean oil, corn oil or safflower oil daily as salad dressing or with tomato or fruit juice, (5) include 2 to 4 tablespoons of whole wheat germ each day, with cereal or salad.

Soybean lecithin is available in capsule, liquid or powder form at health stores everywhere. It is a prime ingredient in Dr. Morrison's *Low-Fat Way to Better Health and Longer Life,* along with sensible weight-reduction and moderate exercise.

Reported Cases:
- **Dr. Morrison reports how 19 elderly patients were placed on this program. All—with one exception—had suffered from a stroke or hardening of the brain arteries. Doctors generally regard such poor souls as hopeless vegetables, he says. All suffered some paralysis of legs, hands or arms, and were weak, listless and de-**

pressed. One had Parkinsonism, the shaking of the hands (tremors) so often seen in the elderly. In 12 weeks they showed striking and dramatic improvement. They were alert, energetic, stronger, some sufficiently well to be discharged from the hospital!

- Dr. Morrison tells of an 83-year-old stroke victim, brought to his office in a wheelchair: "Mrs. A. was too feeble to walk, almost blind, partly deaf, and too weak to feed herself...." Using the Miracle Medicine Food, lecithin, as described in this book, in two months, a miracle happened! "Mrs. A. walked in to see me, under her own power. She was able to see.... Because her hearing had returned, we were able to carry on a conversation." She laughed at having cheated death!

- Dr. Morrison continues: "Take the case of Miss R., a 65-year-old maiden lady who had a stroke (she'd suffered a brain clot due to hardening of the arteries). Her vision was failing and she was partly paralyzed, desperate and depressed...." Using the Miracle Medicine Food, lecithin, as described in his book, he says: "Miss R. recovered much of her muscular powers, her partial paralysis gradually disappeared, and she became a radiant picture of cheerfulness.... Her vision had greatly improved, and when last seen in my office she asked me brightly, 'Doctor, could I go swimming?' I replied, 'Indeed yes, but—no diving!'"

- Lecithin has dramatically reduced some extremely high cholesterol cases. As reported in the *Journal of the Mt. Sinai Hospital*, one woman, age 38, had a reading of 1370! This was reduced to 445 when she took 2½ teaspoonsful of lecithin daily for three months. Other readings of 300 to 600 were cut in half, on about the same dosage in 80 to 12 weeks! A diabetic woman who was very obese reduced her count by 125 points in one and a half months!

- A 60-year-old man with extremely high blood pressure was given an expensive medical treatment which didn't seem to help. After hearing about liquid lecithin, he began taking a tablespoonful daily, and in a matter of weeks his blood pressure dropped over 100 points!

- Mr. H.B. suffered severe angina (heart) attacks, and was told by doctors he had only 10 years to live provided he avoid all strenuous exercise. After reading that lecithin keeps cholesterol liquefied in the system, he began taking one tablespoonful daily. Twenty years later, he reported that he was never troubled with angina again!
- Mrs. U., a housewife of 45, had always been ashamed of fatty spots of yellowish hue that appeared on her skin. Soon after she began adding lecithin to her diet, as prescribed by her doctor, the patches began to disappear. Eventually, they vanished altogether.[2]

Olive Oil Is Healing To The Heart!

Another woman claimed that soaking her feet for ten minutes every day in a hot foot-bath prepared with shavings of castile soap reduced her blood cholesterol. She said, "I know it sounds crazy, but it worked—it really did! The drop in cholesterol was confirmed by a doctor." Castile soap is made with pure olive oil, which has been found to reduce cholesterol by as much as 26 percent. In one study where olive oil is widely used, out of 1,215 men, only 4 cases of heart or artery disease were found in six years.[3]

Honey Is A Fine Heart Stimulant!

Honey is a fine heart stimulant—better than brandy or whiskey, which pep up the heart temporarily, and then wear off. Honey has a long-lasting effect, because of its slow-absorbing sugar, levulose. Many doctors have used honey in heart cases. Dr. G.N.W. Thomas, of Edinburgh, Scotland, in an article in *Lancet* remarked that "in heart weakness I have found honey to have a marked effect in reviving the heart action in keeping patients alive. I had further evidence of this in a recent case of pneumonia. The patient consumed two pounds

---

[2]*The Low-Fat Way to Health and Longer Life,* Ibid.
[3]Richard Lucas, *The Magic of Herbs in Daily Living,* Parker Publishing Co., Inc., 1972.

of honey during the illness; there was an early crisis with no subsequent rise of temperature and an exceptionally good pulse."

Alcohol Is a Miracle Medicine Food That Can Improve Circulation!

Alcohol, used in small or moderate amounts, is indeed a miracle medicine food. Not food in the sense of forming healthy body tissue, says Dr. Morrison,[4] but rather as a stimulant, sedative and pain-reliever. Used in many medicines as a solvent and preservative, it also stimulates the appetite by increasing the flow of gastric juices, relaxes the stomach muscles, open blood vessels and seems helpful to the circulation. In small amounts, it is a mild stimulant to the heart and kidneys, an excellent antiseptic, and is sometimes given intravenously following surgery, to supply a concentrated form of energy.

It opens up and increases the flow of circulation better than any new drug Dr. Morrison has seen. "I have seen and helpfully treated with alcohol many sufferers from arteriosclerosis of the legs who were unable to walk and at times faced gangrene and amputation of the toes or feet," he says.

One patient, Mr. J., 48, was getting severe attacks of angina (chest pain) every time he had lunch and supper, so he stopped eating. After a loss of thirty pounds and a problem of underweight, Dr. Morrison urged him to take one brandy or whiskey before each meal, and to have two glasses of wine at lunch and supper. He tried it. Miraculously, the pain disappeared. Normal weight was restored, he ate his food in a relaxed manner and enjoyed it.

Papaya Is A Heart Food, Too!

Papaya contains an enzyme known as *carpain* which is extremely valuable to the heart. A physician reported the case

---

[4]*The Low-Fat way to Health and Longer Life*, Ibid.

of Dianna B., 30, who, for 26 weeks, had been suffering excruciatingly painful attacks of angina pectoris and had fainting spells. She had been taking as many as a dozen pills a day, and believed the end was near. She was advised to eat nothing but mangos and papayas. In a short time, her pains were completely gone, her heart beat normally, and her health was restored!

Heartbeat Revived With Miracle Medicine Foods!

A reported case[5] is that of Mrs. R. who was in her early 60's and had severe hardening of the arteries, high blood pressure, and almost no heartbeat at all. She was in a semicoma when she was treated. Mrs. R. was so sick, she was given up for lost. She was given an iodine supplement together with B complex vitamins in the form of brewer's yeast three times daily. This was reportedly the only medication she received.

Yet it worked so well her eyelids fluttered open, her blood pressure became normal. She was soon out of bed, able to go about her daily tasks and begin living again!

After she was released from the hospital (where she had been taken as a last and hopeless resort), Mrs. R. continued taking the iodine-vitamin B complex combination every single day. Her hardening of the arteries eased up, her heart was youthful, her skin had a healthy color, her personality was vivacious, and she felt young all over again. Mrs. R. had more than twenty years added to her life (she reached her upper eighties). For her, the aging process had been postponed!

Miracle Medicine Foods Save Victim of Eight Heart Attacks!

Mr. M.A. reports: "Four years ago I was in such bad health that I had very little hope of living much longer. I

---

[5]*The Natural Laws of Healthful Living,* Carlson Wade, Parker Publishing Co., Inc., 1970.

had had eight heart attacks, four of which hospitalized me. One had resulted in an infarction. I could not engage in any extra exertion without having to sit down for a while. I had arthritis so badly that I could not walk without pain. My hands would cramp until the fingers overlapped."

> **Then he discovered Miracle Medicine Foods: "For three years I have taken vitamins A and B complex, together with yeast and liver, about three grams of C each day, kelp, dolomite, bone meal and other calcium capsules, lecithin, pantothenic acid, etc. I can now mow our lawn —and that takes about two hours—walk a vigorous mile, and sleep deeply all night."**

"I also take a mineral complex to get my zinc and extra magnesium," he says. "Another side effect of these vitamins and a healthy diet is improving eyesight. Three years ago my E.E.N.T. specialist told me he would have to remove cataracts from both eyes. The cataracts are gradually disappearing and I can see much better."

No Longer Staggers When She Gets Out of Bed!

Mrs. G.P. writes: "I have a history of rheumatic fever and endocarditis, also hardening of the arteries around the heart which causes angina. This was much worse as shown in (an) EKG taken in the hospital. I had gotten to the place where I staggered when I first got out of bed or when I would get up out of my chair. I'm 72 years old.

"The doctor said to increase my pills for hardening of the arteries from one a day to four a day! I thought I remembered reading about something ... for hardening of arteries and angina ... lecithin, wheat germ, yeast, bone meal and safflower oil. I went to the health food store and stocked up on them. I began taking them every morning with my cereal. ...

"In December just before Christmas I went for my monthly EKG. I asked the doctor how it was and he said, 'It's normal!' "

Excruciating Heart Pain Disappeared—
Claims Miracle Food Better Than Pills!

Mrs. J.M. says: "Four years ago, at age 62, I couldn't walk across the street without terrible chest pain. Excess fluid was causing a heart problem. I had to quit my job and go to a hospital. After a week of many x-rays and cardiograms, I was sent home with a prescription for two kinds of 'water pills.' One pill gave me horrible muscle spasms—such excruciating agony, I'd cry—so I stopped taking it. My chest still hurt. Back at the hospital I had more tests, and no answers. More water pills. Then I heard about vitamin B-6 being good for edema (too much fluid) in pregnant women. I tried it and lost seven or eight pounds within a week! I put my doctor's water pills in the garbage. I've been taking B-6 ever since (plus brewer's yeast, desiccated liver, and vitamins A, B, C, D and E). I can now walk miles, do my own housework and help raise and can our own vegetables. Climbing hills is still hard for me, but I haven't been to another doctor in four years."

Nausea, Dizziness and Tendency
Toward "Little Strokes" Virtually Cured!

Mrs. I.E. reports: "I am 80 years old. About 3 years ago, my tendency toward morning nausea seemed to be getting worse and was accompanied sometimes by dizziness; I had a slight stroke and threatened to have more. About that time, I read somewhere that a dentist was recommending grated citrus peel to his patients and was getting results. The article was brief and did not tell what kind of results. I decided to try the peel anyway, as I had already discovered that bitter foods helped to relieve nausea somewhat. Ever since then, I have been grating the rind of about one-half lemon (or its equivalent in orange or lime peel) into my fruit salad or fruit compote once a day.

"It has practically cured my nausea, dizziness and tendency toward little strokes. I had no idea until four or five months ago what element in the peel was helping me. I ran across a brief statement in the newspaper about the vitamin P in citrus peel being a very important vitamin. It is a tasty addition to my carefully regulated diet. I use a special small grater and grate a little raw carrot after the peel in order to catch it all."

Painful Varicose Veins Gone!

Mrs. N.R. reports: "When I was pregnant with my second son, I developed very painful varicose veins in my left leg. After my son's birth I assumed they were gone. But when I resumed my dance training, I found I was wrong. After four hours on the dance floor my leg would be killing me! So I temporarily gave up dance.

"I started to read a lot and began to realize that what I needed were extra vitamins. Bingo! I put myself on a vitamin regimen with extra B-6, folic acid, and vitamin E. At the same time I got back on the dance floor. Well, it didn't happen overnight, but after two months my legs didn't hurt as much after class. So I increased the E to 400 I.U. daily and three months later I noticed that the veins were gone! No ugly veins bulging on my legs! Even the little 'spider veins' around my ankle were gone!"

Diabetic's Varicose Vein Normal!

Mr. H.M. reports: "Because of a family background of heart trouble and diabetes, I started on vitamin E and other vitamins and minerals some four years ago. Prior to that time I had a case of phlebitis which seemed to have healed normally.

"Recently I noted that the vein in my leg that had been affected began to develop a varicose condition. The vein was enlarged and showed the common dark blue condition associated with this type of problem. This was about two months ago, and at that time I increased my vitamin E intake from 2000 units a day to 3000 units. I also increased my vitamin C from 1000 mg. to 2000 mg. Within two weeks the vein was, and still is, back to normal.

"The one other note on vitamin E is that prior to starting on it I was taking medicine (Orinase) for diabetes. My doctor said I would have to take it the rest of my life, but after a short time of vitamin E I was able to stop the use of it. My fasting blood sugar is always between 85 and 95. My doctor says that it is temporarily abated, but I believe it's the vitamin E."

Vitamin E For Buerger's Disease!

Miss R.S. reports: "A few years ago, I suddenly developed Buerger's Disease in my left foot—the first 3 toes were cyanotic and I had an abscess on the third toe. I had terrific pains in my leg, painful walking, and was unable to sleep. I went to a doctor who wanted to amputate the toes. I refused. After reading about vitamin E, I immediately increased my intake from 800 I.U.'s daily to 1600 and gradually to 2400 I.U.'s a day, along with lecithin granules and 500 mg. of vitamin C—massaged my foot and exercised.

"Within 3 days the pain was almost gone and I was able to sleep and walk better. To say the least, I still have my toes and they look normal in color. I've always had a circulatory problem and 3 years ago dissolved a blood clot in my leg almost overnight with vitamin E. If it wasn't for vitamin E I might be minus 3 toes and who knows, by now, probably part of my foot." (Note: *The International Record of Medicine*, July 1951, reports that of 18 patients with Buerger's Disease treated with vitamin E, 17 were cured!)

Comfrey For Varicose Leg Ulcers!

Mrs. S.W. reports: "What I know about comfrey is too good to keep. My husband had varicose ulcers on his legs. His line of work (years of standing) caused the veins to burst. We doctored at a hospital in Oakland, California, and for two years I used what they gave me, putting it on twice a day, and wrapping with ace-bandages. At the end of two years the ulcers were no better than the day we started.

"Having heard of comfrey being called the miracle herb, I got several big leaves, put them through a juicer, diluted them, put the pulp on some gauze, and used this poultice just one a day. In six weeks my husband had not one ulcer on his legs.

"They were completely healed. We have moved... and have two comfrey plants started already in the garden. I wouldn't be without it."

Phlebitis Victim Back on Her Feet Again!

Ms. H.N. reports: "Up until recently I had so much pain with phlebitis that I was in bed for three months. Then a friend told me about vitamin E and I have been taking 400 mg. daily and now I walk for an hour or more every morning. Then I help at Senior Citizens for four hours, five days a week besides all the other things I do and my legs do not bother me now. I will be 70 years old soon and have more energy than my daughter who is 32. I am so grateful for vitamin E. It has been my life saver!"

Phlebitis Ulcer Heals like Magic!

Ms. V.B. reports: "For many years I had suffered phlebitis which eventually broke down and formed an ulcer, which would heal for a while then break open again and again. After one severe case of infection, I had to have surgery, which helped, but only temporarily. By this time I had a great area of scar tissue which would crack, with the result, further ulceration occurred. My doctor wanted further surgery and skin graft, which I refused.

"I engaged a new doctor; he agreed with me a trial with vitamin E might be of some merit. He put me on 1600 units a day, plus application externally to the affected area. It was like magic. The ulcers healed, the scar tissue became pliable, no further breakage. The bulgy veins flattened down to normal.

"I stayed on vitamin E for six weeks under doctor's supervision. Then decreased to 800 per day for three months. I now continue to take 400 units each day. Never felt better in my life. Considering I'm in my sixties and worked standing on my feet eight hours a day, this was a severe test for any medication.

Phlebitis Relieved, Clot Disappears, Paralysis Avoided!

Mr. D.S. relates how his neighbor developed a clot in his right thigh, which was removed surgically. The operation was a great success, he says. Unfortunately, the man's leg was permanently paralyzed. Then he says: "Last May I served on the election board... and was on my feet practically all (day). By the next morning an alarming blood clot had formed in the femoral vein in my left thigh. The flesh around the vein was red and inflamed. The vein stood out under the skin like a rope on the inside portion of my thigh and was very sore to the touch... I feared that surgery... I had been taking about 1200 I.U. of vitamin E daily, so I decided... to double the dose... and within 24 hours the clot began to disappear. The hard rope-like vein in my thigh had softened. I continued taking 2400 I.U. of vitamin E for several days. After five or six days the clot and inflammation had completely gone. Soon thereafter I had recovered completely."

A Miracle Medicine Food For High Blood Pressure!

Reportedly, hundreds of physicians have found garlic to be the safest, most dependable way to relieve high blood pressure. No one knows exactly why this is so. Some doctors think it dilates (opens) arteries, relieving pressure. Others cite its germicidal power to relieve infections of various kinds, and thereby reduce elevated blood pressure.

Blood pressure is definitely reduced, however. Doctors report—in case after case tested—such symptoms as weakness, dizziness, throbbing headaches, ringing in the

ears, angina-like chest pains, shortness of breath, backaches, numbness, or tingling sensations—all relieved quickly and easily!

In fact, garlic seems to fulfill all the requirements of a perfect therapeutic agent to reduce blood pressure:

1. It is absolutely safe!
2. No bad after effects, no limit to dosage have been found!
3. Blood pressure is reduced gradually—over a period of time—without a sudden drop that could shock the system!
4. It will not interfere with any other medication you may be taking, under a doctor's care!
5. In almost every case tested, it has relieved weakness, dizziness, headaches, ringing ears, chest pain, and annoying gas pains!
6. Good results may be obtained regardless of age or condition!
7. It is easy to take, in odor-free tablet form!

Currently, garlic tablets and capsules, available without prescription at health stores everywhere, are widely used by doctors for reducing high blood pressure and relieving its symptoms.

High blood pressure is extremely dangerous because, first, these symptoms are not always present—many sufferers are completely unaware they have it—and second, it will almost always lead to heart, vein and artery trouble in the form of a stroke, a clot, a hemorrhage, kidney failure, heart failure or sudden death, if not controlled.

One thing should be clear, however—garlic is not a cure for high blood pressure; it merely relieves the pressure and strain on heart, veins and arteries, plus any other annoying symptoms, which may return when garlic therapy is stopped. However, prolonged use of garlic in many cases has tended to permanently lower high blood pressure!

Lowers High Blood Pressure, Raises Low Blood Pressure—In as Little As An Hour!

Kristine Nolfi, a Danish physician and naturopath, and author of *My Experiences With Living Foods*, states: "Garlic ... lowers too high blood pressure and raises one which is too low..." French scientist Pouillard found this to be true. He claimed a decided drop in pressure within an hour after the first administration of garlic. He also noted that it causes low blood pressure to rise.

Good Results May Be Obtained Regardless Of Age Or Condition!

G. Piotrowski, visiting lecturer and member of the faculty of medicine at the University of Geneva, believed that garlic lowers blood pressure by dilating the blood vessels. In an article in *Praxis*, July 1, 1948, he reports using garlic on about 100 patients. He began by giving fairly large doses of oil of garlic, which he gradually diminished over a period of three weeks. He then continued with small, intermittent doses for the balance of the treatment (he does not say how long this lasted). During this time, patients went about their daily lives as usual. In 40 percent of the cases, blood pressure dropped two centimeters.

This expected drop, he says, generally takes place after about a week of treatment. Symptoms such as headaches, dizziness, ringing in the ears, angina-like pains and pains between the shoulder blades began to disappear in three to five days after the garlic treatment began. In cases of headaches, especially, 80 percent of those treated reported relief. Patients found that they could think much more clearly and concentrate on their jobs.

Good results may be obtained, regardless of age or condition, he notes. Old or young, high or low, the blood pressure tends to normalize. Garlic causes a drop in blood pressure, in most cases, he states—and whether or not results are completely normal, he says the use of garlic is justified by the relief it brings for uncomfortable symptoms of high blood pressure. He concludes by recommending that many more M.D.'s begin immediately to use garlic therapy in treating high blood pressure.

Blood Pressure Normalized!

One man, Gerald R., reports using garlic and rutin (found in buckwheat cakes) and eliminating salt to lower his blood pressure from 170 to 120/70. Another, Mr. Ted S. reports:

> "I had part of a bottle of garlic perles sitting on the refrigerator for several months and hadn't taken but a few of them on occasion. Nevertheless, after reading about all the benefits to be derived from garlic I decided to give them a try. My reason was mainly to lower my blood pressure, which a doctor referred to as the high side of normal. After taking the perles for about five weeks, I found that my blood pressure had gone down to 126/90 after being about 140/90 for quite some time. Just to make sure I had the woman in the clinic take it a second time and it came out the same."

"As an added bonus," he says, "taking garlic perles for only one week brought an end to a type of diarrhea and colitis which I had had continually for three and one-half years! This cure was a complete surprise to me!"

Dangerously High Blood Pressure Is Normalized!

"Rejoice with me!" says Mr. D.G. "My blood pressure is now completely normal, thanks to garlic! I'm in my forties. Six months ago I had my yearly physical. I had high blood pressure of 190 over 90 and lots of weight. Advised to lose weight, I did not. But I did get interested in garlic as a means to bring down my blood pressure and started taking daily one garlic capsule.

"Last week I was asked to give a pint of blood for a friend in the local hospital and when they took my blood pressure it was a mere 130/75! And I haven't lost an ounce of weight so it must be the garlic as I haven't changed one thing except that.

"One thing I do want to impress," Mr. D.G. concludes, "is that I was meticulous in taking the capsule, one every day without fail."

Garlic In Foot and Hand Baths!

Finally—and this is a recipe not to be taken internally—garlic has been used in the form of foot and hand baths, for relief of high blood pressure, in this remedy for hypertension used by famed herbalist, Maurice Mességué:

Garlic (one large crushed head)
Single-seed hawthorn (blossom—one handful)
Greater celandine (leaves, semi-fresh if possible—one handful)
Common bloom (flowers—one handful)

Follow the basic instructions on page 37 of Chapter 2 for preparation of this foot and hand bath, and use as often as needed. Mességué claims that he has had 60 percent success with it (30 percent cured, 30 percent greatly relieved, and 40 percent unknown—meaning the patients failed to keep him posted on the results). Mességué advises that a diet prescribed by the doctor in charge should be followed.[6]

(Such a diet usually includes several glasses of water a day, and plenty of bulk foods—fresh fruits and vegetables—to avoid constipation. Acid-forming foods are avoided, as well as sharp cheeses, spices and alcohol. Little or no salt is used, and plenty of rest and relaxation are recommended.)

---

[6]Reprinted with permission of Macmillan Publishing Co., Inc., from *Of Men and Plants* by Maurice Mességué. Copyright © 1972 by Weidenfeld & Nicolson Ltd. Copyright © 1973 by Macmillan Publishing Co., Inc.

Garlic—The Miracle Heart Food!

The French scientist Pouillard found that garlic has a remarkable effect on the heart. In cases of diseases of the heart and the aorta (the great artery that arises from the heart) garlic juice taken over a period of ten days produced a definite improvement in both rhythm and heart action, he stated. It relieved dizziness, angina-like pains and backaches in three to five days.

Dr. L.J. Maisonneuvre, in Marraine, France says: "Garlic dissolves the crystals, the accumulation of which causes hardening of the arteries. It lowers the blood pressure, accelerates and regulates the blood circulation by stimulating the heart muscles and acts as a blood purifier at the same time."

"Therefore," says Dr. Maisonneuvre, "it gives excellent results in a number of troubles due to deficient circulation... like varicose veins, piles, rheumatism, etc."

A Scientific Breakthrough!

In 1961, the Japanese scientist Fujiwara discovered that the sulfur substance in garlic called allicin, speeds the absorption of vitamin B-1 (thiamin) in the body, according to the *Pakistan Medical Times*, May 16, 1961. This vitamin is of extreme importance in heart disorders.

Experts cite this as a major breakthrough. Ordinarily, they say, vitamin B-1 is not easily digestible—whether from foods or food supplements—and gets through the intestinal wall slowly and in reduced amounts. But when combined with garlic into a substance called allithiamin, blood concentration of vitamin B-1 increased TENFOLD to a level heretofore impossible to achieve except by liquid injection!

In addition, garlic contains manganese—a mineral needed by humans in trace amounts—which keeps excessive amounts of vitamin B-1 from overreacting in the body.

Effect of B-1 On Enlarged Heart!

The most essential items for "heart food" are oxygen and lactic acid. The body uses oxygen to burn lactic acid in enormous quantities in the heart muscles. Vitamin B-1 is the catalyst or stimulant (like a match) that causes this to happen.

Without sufficient vitamin B-1, the heart muscles become weak and enlarged. Proof of this is the fact that in Asia, where diets often lack this vitamin, enlarged hearts (almost double the size of a normal heart) are quite common.

Dr. S. Weiss, of Harvard Medical School, proved that myocardial heart failure (weakness of the heart muscle) stems from lack of vitamin B-1 by showing that, even if the heart is greatly enlarged, it can be reduced in size in 48 hours with large doses of vitamin B-1!

Medical Recommendations!

In the *Texas State Medical Journal* (May 1943), L.P. Hightower advocates the administration of vitamin B-1 to all patients with indefinite heart symptoms, especially in cases of known deficiency. He recommends injections of 100 milligrams of thiamin per day, along with a diet high in vitamin B rich foods. This, he says, is usually followed by a prompt improvement. The size of the heart is reduced and improvements appear in electrocardiograms.

A Miracle Recovery From Heart Failure!

The annals of medical literature tell of a 72-year-old man, George S., who seemed to be suffering from bronchitis and failure of the right side of the heart. He received antibiotics and cardiac therapy to no avail.

Further tests revealed he was suffering from lack of vitamin B-1! He was immediately given 100 mg. injections of B-1 plus B-1 tablets. Dramatic and early relief followed!

The heart symptoms ceased and the patient was soon walking!

Strangely enough, George S. showed none of the usual signs of B-1 deficiency (loss of appetite, numbness and tingling in toes and feet, stiffness in ankles, pains in legs). It may be, said the doctor, that right heart failure in some cases is due to poor storage capacity in the body for vitamin B-1 and also a diet deficient in B vitamins.

Foods rich in B vitamins (it is inadvisable to consume B-1 alone, except on advice of a physician) include brewer's yeast, organ meats, and dessicated liver. Trace amounts of vitamin B-1 are present in garlic. Garlic's major value, however, is that it speeds the body's absorption of this vitamin tenfold!

Garlic Dissolves Cholesterol!

Two Indian doctors, Drs. Bordia and Bansal, reporting in the December 29, 1973, issue of *The Lancet*, the British medical journal, state that garlic has a "very significant protective action" against cholesterol and other fats in the bloodstream—and also reduces the tendency of the blood to form dangerous clots. A recent news item summarizes these findings as follows:

Claims Eating Garlic Can Help Prevent Arteries From Clogging!

Eating garlic may help prevent diseased arteries.
Medical tests have shown that the pungent root has a "very signficant protective action" in limiting the effects of fat blood coagulation, said Drs. Arun Bordia and H.C. Bansal of R.N.T. Medical College, Udaipur, India.
Reporting in the British medical journal *Lancet*, the doctors said the blood of 10 patients clotted more slowly when they ate garlic with fatty food than when they ate it without garlic.
They said this meant garlic could slow down the buildup

of fatty deposits on artery walls and help prevent the arteries from clogging.

—*National Enquirer*, March 17, 1974

Specifically, 100 grams of butter (nearly a quarter of a pound) were added to a regular meal which the test patients ate. Three hours later, they averaged a blood cholesterol count of 237.4 milligrams percent.

When the juice or oil extracted from 50 grams of garlic was added to the identical meal, after three hours the blood cholesterol count was only 212.7 milligrams percent. It was found that garlic oil alone has the full effect—whether taken as pure oil, as garlic juice or in whole garlic.

In addition, garlic oil reduced the level of fibrogen (a clotting factor) in the blood. A meal containing butter resulted in a fibrogen level of 320.9 milligrams percent—in three hours. When garlic was added to the same meal, the blood level of fibrogen, three hours later, was 256.4.

Garlic in both cases actually brought the levels of cholesterol and fibrogen *below their fasting levels*.

"Pinging" In Head Relieved!

Suzy N., 58, a housewife and mother, began suffering from an annoying "ping" in her temples. It would come like a "shot," or perhaps one or two "stabbing pains," and go away just as fast—sometimes on the right side of her head and sometimes on the left. It even seemed to happen when she was relaxing, perhaps writing a letter or reading. At first the attacks were few, once every couple of weeks or so. They frightened her more than anything else. She feared a cerebral hemorrhage, like a friend her age had had, or hardening of the arteries. Then the attacks became more frequent, practically every single day. Along with this she experienced a ringing in the ears, that did not go away; a constant ringing, buzzing, whistling sound, day and night, that made it very difficult to concentrate.

A drug was prescribed that she later found out was for "peripheral vascular disease, vascular spasm" and an ear condition. The literature stated that it was a vasodilator (capable of dilating blood vessels) and contained nicotinyl alcohol in a tartrate salt. Almost as much as the head pain, she feared the side effects, which including flushing, stomach upset, rashes and allergic reactions.

Instead she decided to try garlic. She had heard that garlic had a good effect on veins and arteries, that it was a natural dilator—letting more blood through—and could dissolve fatty deposits on artery walls, preventing clogging. Also, it would be extremely healing to the nerves due to its vitamin B-1 or thiamin-boosting factor. It was reportedly safe and long-lasting, with no bad side-effects. It was also inexpensive and easily obtained.

Since using garlic daily, the "pinging" sensations, the frequent pain and discomfort, have completely disappeared. The "buzzing" sensation is gone, and there are no flushing, stomach upset or rashes to contend with.

Garlic and Hardening of The Arteries!

In view of the research by Dr. Maisonneuvre, who states that "Garlic dissolves the crystals, the accumulation of which causes hardening of the arteries," as well as the work of Drs. Arun Bordia and H.C. Bansal, who stated that garlic has a "very protective action" against cholesterol and other fats in the bloodstream, which could prevent arteries from clogging —the following remedies listed by Maurice Mességué, in *Of Men and Plants,* should prove of interest:

ARTERIOSCLEROSIS (hardening of the arteries)
   Garlic (two large crushed heads)
   Single-seed hawthorn (blossom—one handful)
   Greater celandine (leaves and stems semi-fresh if possible—one handful)
   Common broom (flowers and young shoots—one handful)

This may be prepared—and used in foot- and hand-baths —following the basic instructions on page 37 of Chapter 2. In addition, follow a diet recommended by your doctor, says Mességué.

ARTERITIS (inflammation of the arteries)
  Garlic (one large crushed head)
  Artichoke (leaves—one handful)
  Single-seed hawthorn (blossom—one handful)
  Sage (flowers and leaves—one handful)
  Thyme (leaves and flowers—one handful)

Once again, this may be prepared—for use in foot- and hand-baths—following the basic instructions in Chapter 2. Mességué claims an 85 percent success rate in healing inflammation of the arteries with this method (15 percent cured, 70 percent greatly relieved, 15 percent unknown). He states, however, that since inflammation of the arteries may stem from many causes, this remedy may bring relief, but is not necessarily a cure.[7]

Massage Can Relieve Heart!

The heart may be relieved and healed by massaging various nerve ends on the hands and feet. These nerves are located on the left foot, under the third, fourth and fifth toes, and on the left hand, under the last two fingers. Massage the pads at the base of these fingers and toes, until any tenderness disappears. Massaging the little toe or finger on the left hand or foot can relieve heart pain in seconds, say experts, and can be miracle medicine food for your heart!

> No matter what the nature of the trouble is, says one expert, the heart can be aided with this secret. We are told how a man prevented a heart attack in seconds with this method! Almost immedately the pain disappeared and never returned. An elderly bedridden woman with trembling hands and difficult breathing had to be helped up steps. With this miracle medicine food she felt immediate relief, and walked rapidly in a week without help!

---

[7]Reprinted with Permission of Macmillan Publishing Co., Inc., from *Of Men and Plants* by Maurice Mességué. Copyright © 1972 by Weidenfeld & Nicholson Ltd. Copyright © 1973 by Macmillan Publishing Co., Inc.

This miracle medicine food for your body requires no expense, no special equipment, and can be used by anyone in perfect safety, says this expert. It has brought relief to countless suffering people, when all hope had seemingly been lost, can cure specific ailments, and restores organs to perfect health, says this expert.

Emergency Heart Attack Relief!

Along with nerve massage, which can prevent a heart attack in seconds, according to experts, strong mental commands can wall out pain to an astonishing degree. One man suffered an excruciating heart attack, so bad he was given only a slight chance of survival. His wife told him to use this method, which not only relieved his pain, but his recovery was rapid and dramatic. The attending doctor never saw anything like it! In one month, he was back at work! Mental commands can be miracle medicine food, restoring perfect health to the heart and circulatory system, repairing any damage done by previous heart attacks, and miracuolusly speeding up the healing so that injuries vanish in an amazingly short time, says one expert, adding that with a doctor's help they'll fully prepare you to handle any heart attack emergency! Here, at your fingertips in this chapter, is the instant relief for heart, veins and high blood pressure!

4

Miracle Medicine Foods For Liver And Gall Bladder Problems!

Gall bladder symptoms include indigestion, gas, a feeling of fullness, nausea, constipation, eye problems (including spots before the eyes, cataracts), and swollen ankles. Other symptoms include inability to digest fats, sharp stabbing pains, pressure under the ribs, a frequent belching bitter taste, heart attack symptoms, cold sweats, jaundice, itching red skin on the back, clay-colored or dry, hard stools (same as for liver trouble), varicose veins, phlebitis, and hemorrhoids. Sufferers complain of headaches and are frequently irritable. These symptoms can be relieved a number of ways:

1. Gall bladder symptoms can be relieved by surgery, but frequently return—even after removal of the organ!
2. Many gall bladder victims fail to eat breakfast, but doctors recommend a good high fiber breakfast to start the bile juice flowing. Drs. Neil Painter and Kenneth Heaton of England state that food like bran "sweeps the degenerated bile salts out of the colon and the vast majority of patients report relief of symptoms."
3. Another doctor[1] claims you can usually get a lazy gall

---

[1] John E. Eichenlaub, *A Minnesota Doctor's Home Remedies for Common and Uncommon Ailments.* (Prentice-Hall, 1960.)

bladder into action by simply taking one or two tablespoons of olive oil before each meal. This starts the flow of bile before the rest of the food enters the stomach. You may get a bit more indigestion, he says, for the first few days, but you should see marked improvement inside two weeks.

4. A low-fat (*not* a no-fat) diet helps ward off further attacks, says this doctor. Some fat is necessary to keep bile juices flowing and to dissolve vitamins A, D, E and K which cannot be absorbed without fat. However, fried foods, pork, rich pastries and gravies, etc., must go. Replace cream with half-and-half, avoid whipping cream and keep butter down to a few pats a day. Eat plenty of lean broiled or boiled meat, vegetables and fruit, he says.

5. Nutrition experts have stated that foods such as yeast, nuts, and unrefined grains increase the production of lecithin, which breaks up or liquefies gall stones. The English medical journal *Lancet* (May 26, 1956) says: "Two preventive measures for gallstones are sunflower seeds and brewer's yeast." Beet tops have also been recommended for speeding the flow of bile.

6. Large meals should be avoided, say experts, and one doctor[2] states: "Studies indicate the gallbladder sufferers seldom put water on the table and drank much less fluid than other people." Water is, therefore, recommended.

7. For gas upset due to a sluggish liver or gallbladder, eliminating fatty foods from your diet, including fried eggs, beans, pork, butter, margarine, milk, and cream may eliminate the problem. In addition, don't eat for at least four hours before retiring. Charcoal tablets (available at many health food stores) can also bring relief.

8. Walking or moderate exercise is also recommended. Gall bladder sufferers are frequently inactive, causing stasis in the bile duct.

---

[2] John E. Eichenlaub, *Op. cit.*

Gallstones Can Be Passed!

Gallstones can be passed, unnoticed, if they are small enough. But if they become lodged in the bile duct, they can cause blockage and acute pain, radiating from the right side to the shoulder, with nausea and cold sweats, that may subside and return, from time to time.

If your doctor has determined with X-rays that your gallstones are small enough to be passed without getting stuck, an old folk remedy for passing them—occasionally recommended by doctors—is to mix half a cup of olive oil with half a cup of lemon or grapefruit juice, stir, drink and go to bed. You may experience nausea. In the morning, drink something hot and you may pass the stones from your bowels.

Another method is to fast for two days, drinking apple juice at two-hour intervals, and use the preceding method on the second night. This is said to dissolve the stones and cleanse the bladder too. One doctor says that three tablespoons of undiluted, unsweetened lemon juice, fifteen to thirty minutes before breakfast daily, for a week, is so powerful that it will stimulate, purge and empty the gallbladder.

Gallstones Can Be Dissolved (in as little at 24 hours)!

Gallstones can be prevented with soybean lecithin, according to Dr. R.K. Tompkins of Ohio State University College of Medicine. It appears to liquefy the main substance—cholesterol—of which human gallstones are composed!

In *Common and Uncommon Uses of Herbs for Healthful Living*, Richard Lucas reports that olive oil is a valuable preventive against gallstones. The oil causes strong healthy contractions of the gall bladder, greatly favoring complete emptying, and can be regarded as a very good gall bladder tonic. Olive oil also seems to melt gallstones. He says that in 1893 an experiment was re-

ported by Dr. E.M. Brockbank, in which a gallstone lost 68 percent of its weight when immersed in pure olive oil.

Chamomile tea has long been known to dissolve gallstones. Nicholas Culpepper wrote: "That it is excellent for the stone, appears in this which I have tried, viz.,—that a stone that hath been taken out of the body of a man, being wrapped in chamomile, will in time dissolve, and in a little time, too."

Reported Cases:
- In one reported case, two gallstones were placed in a glass of chamomile tea. The next day the stones were in four pieces. In five days they were like gravel. In ten days they were completely dissolved!
- M.C. writes: "A number of years ago a complete physical by a very reputable clinic showed I had gallstones. I saw the X-ray, and there were five of various sizes. Through friends... I learned how to get rid of them. For three days drink good organic apple juice. Do not eat or drink anything else, except at the end of the second and third day drink half a cup olive oil with half a cup apple juice. The gallstones passed on the fourth day. Several years later I had X-rays... and the doctor reported no signs of gallstones."
- D.R. writes: "My sister was scheduled for surgery after being told she had gallstones. A relative advised her to wait and try the juice of half a lemon placed in a small wine glass and float four tablespoons of olive oil on top to take one hour before breakfast each day. She did this for about six months and found no need for surgery."
- Mrs. F.C. reports: "My husband and I both were bothered with gall bladder pains for about a year. When talking with a naturopath he told us to take, first thing in the morning before anything else, one ounce of vegetable oil and follow with four ounces of grapefruit juice... we substituted four ounces of water with a teaspoon of vinegar. We were never bothered again with any pains... a year later we ran out of oil and

did not use any for three weeks. The gall bladder pains returned, but immediately left as soon as we started the oil and vinegar water again. Now another year has gone and we are still not bothered with gall bladder pains."
• R.K. states: "I have found that very often both gallstones and kidney stones can be 'dissolved' if the diet is adequate in magnesium. My daughter, at age 25, was having an attack of gallstone colic every week or so. After getting her on a natural foods diet, and taking six to eight dolomite tablets daily, she has had no more attacks in the past six years. Other doctors who saw her at the time recommended surgery to remove the gallbladder." (R.K. is an osteopathic doctor.)

More Miracle Medicine Foods For Liver And Gall Bladder!

Dr. Grume, according to the *United States Dispensatory*, uses radish juice in the treatment of cholelithiasis—gall bladder stones. To prevent gallstones, he uses the juice of the crushed roots in doses of two to four ounces. We are told by T.H. Bartram that dandelion coffee not only prevents formation of gallstones, but that 'Hepatitis, or inflammation of the liver, and jaundice, when uncomplicated, readily yield to (it).'[3] Swinburne Clymer, M.D., says dandelion has a beneficial influence on the biliary organs, "removing torpor and engorgement of the liver as well as of the spleen."[4] And *raw carrot juice* has apparently cured the incurable!

Reported Cases:
• We are told of a woman with splenic leukemia, a blood ailment so serious, doctors say it is invariably fatal. She was horribly thin and emaciated, with advanced arthritis and intestinal failure. Yet she recovered completely on raw carrot juice. Today she is quite active and

---

[3]*Health from Herbs*, June 1953.
[4]*Nature's Healing Agents* (Quakertown, Pa.; The Humanitarian Society, Reg., 1960).

healthy, with a full-time job, and seems to be immune to colds!
- Around the turn of the century, a doctor wrote: Fifteen years ago I was afflicted with the liver complaint. I used all my skills trying to cure it, but failed." Then he discovered dandelion root, "taking a teacupful of a strong decoction of it twice a day." He claimed: "In almost every instance I have succeeded in restoring those who have used this plant," including himself!

For gall bladder relief, Dr. Jon Evans of England has reported excellent results in countless cases with extract of the herb greater celandine (10 to 12 drops in a glass of water after each meal) with a diet of fresh fruits and vegetables, lean meat, and no sweets, starches, fried foods, eggs or fat, and dandelion coffee instead of pure coffee.[5]

Sage tea has a sedative effect (a fourteenth-century writer claimed that it cured his palsy: "My hand is as steady as it was at fifteen"), is antiseptic, and purifies the liver and kidneys, according to Father Kneipp, the famous European herbalist.

Rose petals contain malic and tartaric acids, said to be of great value in dissolving out gallstones and gravel from the urinary organs. The dried petals and leaves are often used —with peppermint, lemon peel, and linden leaves—as a tea substitute. This is reportedly helpful also in cases of stomach upset.

Liver Functions Explained!

Basically the liver has two main functions: it manufactures digestive enzymes, and it also acts as a filter between the intestine and the heart. It detoxifies the many "poisons" which we take into our digestive tracts each day, such as nicotine, caffeine, and tannic acid (from tea)—traps and changes them into harmless compounds. The liver cells also catch bacilli and digest them to protect the blood stream. It

---

[5]*Health from Herbs.* September-October 1967.

processes waste nitrogen in the body into urea for excretion, and produces red blood cells.

The Effect of Garlic On Liver Disturbances!

Garlic's major value in liver disorders is its power to detoxify putrefactive bacteria in the intestines (see Chapter 8), and thereby give the liver a rest. It is a proven stimulator of gastric juices (see Chapter 7), which help digestion, and an aid to increased and vigorous blood circulation through the liver.

It is claimed that a teaspoon of garlic mixed with a tablespoon of olive oil or soybean oil, taken at night, will liven up the liver and so rejuvenate it that the skin of the body will glow with renewed activity. Users say it is indeed a miracle vegetable!

Kristine Nolfi, M.D., in her book *My Experiences With Living Food,* states that if garlic is not tolerated it is because of a deficiency in the digestive organs—especially the liver. A stomach or a liver in good condition, she says, will never rebel against an element as natural and beneficial as garlic.

Liver Ailments Relieved!

In his autobiography, *Of Men and Plants,* Maurice Mességué tells about his father. Peasants from miles around—and even the local doctor—consulted Mességué's father, Camille, because of his knowledge of healing plants. The most common complaints, says Mességué, were liver disorders, "because people drank too much and ate such heavy food." And the prime ingredient we find listed for liver and gall bladder trouble is garlic.

Pain Vanishes In 30 Minutes!

"The first time I saw him heal anyone," says Mességué, "it was a neighbor, a man I knew well and whom I saw regularly morning and evening as he passed by. One Monday on his way home he came into our big kitchen bent double: 'Camille, d'you think any of your plants might do me some good? I've got a kind of stabbing pain just here,' indicating his right side.

"That's your liver."

"My father took down some bottles from over the fireplace and mixed several liquids in a bowl. He then made a compress by folding a small piece of flannel, soaked it in the liquid and placed it on the man's side. Within half an hour the pains had gone and his face was no longer screwed up out of all recognition as it had been. . . . It was a miracle!"[6]

Remedy For Liver and Gall Bladder Trouble!

Mességué states that since diseases or disorders of the liver stem from different causes, this preparation only soothes the effects: attacks of pain, digestive troubles, nausea. It may be considered as an excellent basic and general treatment, he says, but for all diseases of the liver it is important to follow a suitable diet prescribed by a doctor.

Garlic (one crushed head)
Milfoil (flowers—one handful)
Artichoke (leaves—one handful)
Greater celandine (leaves and stems, semi-fresh if possible—one handful)
Succory, or chicory (grated roots—one handful)
Hedge-bindweed (flowers and leaves—one handful)
Sage (leaves—one handful)

The basic instructions on page 37, Chapter 2, should be followed. Use either as a foot or hand bath—or as a poultice —but DO NOT EAT. To make a poultice, chop kale and cabbage leaves. Combine with two stiffly beaten egg whites. Wrap this in coarse muslin (linen is not porous enough).

---

[6]Reprinted with permission of Macmillan Publishing Co., Inc., from *Of Men and Plants* by Maurice Mességué. Copyright © 1972 by Weidenfeld & Nicolson Ltd. Copyright © 1973 by Macmillan Publishing Co., Inc.,

Coat this poultice with a small liqueur-glass full of the basic preparation, and apply directly to the skin, on your right side.[7]

More Cases Relieved[8]

Later, when Mességué was a schoolmaster, he found one of his students doubled up with pain. His face was deathly pale. Mességué asked what the matter was. The student pointed to his liver. "At six o'clock I applied a poultice which he kept on all night," says Mességué, "and by the next morning the pain had gone completely."

In another testimonial to the effectiveness of Mességué's garlickly remedy for liver trouble, Mr. Alexander Thomas, the Advocate General of Lyon, gave this sworn statement: "Mességué . . . cured me of a liver disease when I had been given up by the orthodox medical profession."

Gall Bladder Symptoms Relieved!

When Jessica D. was having gall bladder symptoms, a friend suggested she try the Mességué remedy, which had been previously prepared. She was skeptical, but it was a Sunday afternoon, the druggist was closed, and there was no more of the antispasmodic drug the doctor had prescribed in the house.

She leaned against the wall in deathly agony, with stabbing pains in her back, and on her right side, that seemed to grip and seize and shake her in awful spasmodic convulsions from which there was no relief. She complained of extreme nausea, a feeling of pressure up under her ribs, and a frequent belching bitter taste.

A poultice was quickly prepared, over which a small liqueur glass full of the basic preparation was poured, and applied to her side. Within minutes, the pains subsided, and she began to breathe easier. She was told of garlic's powerful penetrative action, its ability to increase circulation and reduce catarrhal swelling of the biliary tract, its mild diuretic and sudorific (sweat inducing) qualities—reducing fever, while

---
[7] *Of Men and Plants,* Maurice Mességué, *Ibid.*
[8] Mességué, *Op cit.*

helping skin and kidneys to expel poisons—its antibacterial, antispasmodic and carminative effect (ability to relieve gas, bloating), its ability to relieve nausea, cramps, and abdominal complaints.

The friend explained that certain other herbal antispasmodics were included in the recipe, such as sage and greater celandine. Even the cabbage has been known to cleanse the mucous membrane of the stomach and intestines, and was used as a near cure-all by Roman physicians for headache, colic, deafness, drunkenness, insomnia and internal ulcers.

Jessica D. was shown how to prepare this remedy herself in foot- and hand-baths, for welcome relief. "The palms of the hands and the soles of the feet are especially sensitive and receptive," says Mességué. "The curative powers of treatments by osmosis are now scientifically explained and accepted." Most importantly, because this garlic preparation is only applied externally—and never eaten, as Mességué points out, it is absolutely safe.

Remedy for a Sluggish Liver!

In *Old Fashioned Health Remedies That Work Best* (Parker Publishing Co., Inc., 1977), L.L. Schneider, D.C., N.D., says that a meat and grape juice diet will relieve a sluggish liver, with pain or tenderness on the right side. White chicken meat, without the skin, and lean meats (especially steak or veal), are recommended. These should be baked, broiled or stewed. Any grape juice may be used, but the easily recognized purple Concord grape is preferred. Grapes help combat liver disorders, jaundice, and stimulate bile flow (they also help burn off excess fat), he says, adding: "If you have acute problems because of your liver, I would make the meat and grape juice diet your exclusive bill of fare—that's right—three times a day. If you just want to be kind to your liver, have an occasional meat and grape juice meal." Diabetics may not be able to use this method, and should check with their doctor first, he says.

Liver and Gall Bladder Pains Relieved In Minutes!

By massaging the outer edge of each hand, near the base of the small finger—massaging out any tenderness there—you can stimulate a sluggish liver and gall bladder, say experts, and pain may be relieved with steady pressure. The same thing can be accomplished by pressing the pad just under the little toe on each foot.

This simple method has relieved liver and gall bladder pain in minutes, and can be miracle medicine food for your body! There are many cases where massage has saved people from having a gall bladder operation, with the stones seeming to vanish after a short time, says one expert!

Some people experience 10 to 12 bowel movements in one day, says this expert, as the liver releases poisons and is cleansed and rejuvenated. One woman with gallstones, was having terrible seizures every few minutes. With this miracle medicine food, she felt immediate relief, and said it was as if a huge wave of pain had lifted! Another woman says that during a gall bladder attack, she tried this miracle medicine food, and her headache and pain disappeared in a matter of minutes! Another man says he tried it, and his gall bladder pains were relieved almost at once! Here is instant relief for liver and gall bladder problems!

5

Miracle Medicine Foods For Kidney, Bladder And Urinary Problems!

Large urate stones (stones caused by excessive uric acid) found in the urinary tract can be dissolved through the simple ingestion of lemon juice, says Dr. Bertrand Bibus, chief urologist, Kaiser Franz Joseph Hospital, Vienna.

He says that such stones have been dissolved by having patients drink the juice of 1 or 2 lemons a day. It was effective in about 50 percent of all cases of large urate stones. "Where small urate stones occur chronically," Dr. Bibus says, "the symptoms, as well as the formation of new stones, cease immediately upon institution of this therapy."

Other common foods that have been used for relief of kidney, bladder and urinary problems include asparagus, beets, black-eyed pea hulls, carrots, cherry juice, cornsilk tea, cranberries, garlic, kidney beans, onions, parsley, radishes, sage tea, and watermelon.

Dr. Ramm's Wonder Cure For Kidneys!

Remarkable permanent cures for kidney and bladder trouble have been achieved with water in which the pods of kidney beans have been cooked. This was discovered by Dr.

Ramm, of Preetz, Germany, around the turn of the century, and reported by him—after 25 years of research.

> Dr. Ramm had been treating a woman for dropsy (accumulation of fluid in the tissues) following a valvular disease of the heart. Nothing worked. Suddenly, while making his rounds one day, he discovered that her swelling was gone! She told him she had accidentally drunk a glass of kidney bean water, and began passing large amounts of crystal clear urine—it happened every time she tried it. After three weeks of this her dropsy was gone!

Just to make sure, she continued drinking the kidney pod tea for a few weeks, then stopped. The condition never returned. Dr. Ramm said she was as healthy as a woman can be. Dr. Ramm tried it on other patients. In all cases of heart disease and other ailments, large quantities of clear urine were passed, and long-standing cases of dropsy were *cured in a matter of days, and stayed cured!*

He found that kidney blockage of long duration was completely cured with bean pod water, and that bleeding from any part of the urinary system was quickly halted! Stones and gravel were rapidly dissolved, and did not return! Diseases of the bladder and ureter were cured! Rheumatism and acute gout vanished! Even some cases of diabetes were cured! In severe cases, it took longer—but it worked if used faithfully! Dr. Ramm called it his "wonder cure!"

In some cases, the kidney bean water caused nausea, in which case Dr. Ramm gave it in enemas instead (a half pint with a teaspoon of salt, every two to four hours)—and the results were just as good as the drink. In fact, the enema seemed to halt the convulsions of uremia, releasing large amounts of water.

Around the same time Dr. Ramm was experimenting with this kidney treatment, Dr. Isenburg of Hamburg was obtaining similar results, as reported by one of Isenberg's patients:

> "About nine years ago, in 1897, I began to suffer from a very disagreeable feeling of pressure in the region of

the bladder, which increased to an intense pain through excitement or psychic depression. In the course of the next few years this state very slowly became worse, until in 1906 violent pains appeared in the right ureter. At the same time the pain in the bladder suddenly increased considerably. My physician diagnosed an inflammation of both organs, but none of those I consulted were able to give any relief.

"The urine showed pus, sometimes in considerable quantities. In 1905, sometimes before these last symptoms developed, other had appeared which consisted of severe pains in the small of the back. They tormented me constantly, and often I could not fall asleep. Cold rubs and liniments only brought a temporary improvement.

"The pains constantly increased during the spring of 1906 and muscular rheumatism set in. This was so violent that I could hardly wash myself in the morning and evening. Rubbings with water and plasters hardly brought any relief. These various ailments finally became so very bad that I was never free from pains; and they increased constantly in violence.

"At this time—in the summer of 1906—the tea of ripe bean pods was recommended to me.... So I sent for five pounds of bean pods. I began the treatment according to directions. I did not have to wait long for results; large masses of uric acid crystals and albuminous matter were excreted, and that initiated a decrease of pain in the bladder and kidneys. The pain in the bladder disappeared entirely in about three weeks, the muscular rheumatism also diminished in the next few weeks, and disappeared entirely in seven or eight weeks.

"I was soon entirely free from my very great sufferings and have not had any trouble since, as I have been using the tea off and on. The enormous excretion of uric acid crystals during the use of the tea was really remarkable (they often covered the bottom of the night vessel)."

Dr. Ramm said that bean pod water must be freshly made and taken the same day as it is prepared. If more than 24 hours old when used, he reported, it causes diarrhea. Dr.

Ramm suggested that beans picked from the garden be used immediately to make a decoction from the sliced pods *without the beans*. (The beans themselves have no value.) Boil two ounces of the pods slowly in four quarts of hot water for four hours. Then filter the liquid through a fine muslin and store in a cool place for eight hours. After eight hours, strain again with muslin—slowly and carefully (too many fibers in the fluid can cause intestinal upset). It is then ready. Dose: one glassful every two hours. Used thus, says Dr. Ramm, the remedy is completely harmless, and can be used indefinitely with excellent results. It drains out pounds of excess fluid!

Reported Results:
- Mrs. B.D. writes: "I developed kidney trouble six weeks (ago). The doctor kept giving me antibiotics but my kidney trouble wouldn't clear up. I went to the third doctor and he told me to come back for tests and x-rays. He found a kidney stone and diabetes. My sugar count was 326. He said I must have an operation if the stone didn't move.... When I got home...I started taking the bean pod tea. I drank a quart a day. Two weeks later when I went back to the doctor my stone was gone and my sugar count was 128. He said 'you're well.' I no longer had a stone nor diabetes. He was as surprised as I. At no time was I given any medication for diabetes."
- Mr. D.S. writes: "My wife has had kidney problems for years...I (prepared a liquid from the plant) taking care to strain and re-strain the fluid, since any extra particles of suspended matter might play havoc with a weaker digestive system. After (letting it stand eight hours), I told my wife to consume an eight-ounce glass every hour. She said the stuff tasted awful and made a lot of faces, but you know what? The concoction worked. Her urine appeared crystal clear after she drank the juice, and she has reported no kidney pain or problems in the kidney area since."
- Mrs. T.D. writes: "I had dropsy for several years and was taking dropsy pills for swelling and fluid.... Then I started cooking these red kidney bean pods, boiling

them (and drinking the water)....I began the treatment according to directions. I did not have to wait long for results. Seems I passed large quantities of urine real often (and some gravel). I continued taking the bean water for about 2½ weeks and within two weeks I had no sign of dropsy. The swelling had left my legs and ankles. The fluid above my stomach had also left."

- Miss K.B. writes: "My urethra had been swollen for years. I've been to Duke Hospital and my own hospital and another one. They cut and treated, but nothing helped. I planted the beans and drank tea made with them for three weeks, and I've never had such results. It took out the swelling all over the body and it was equal to a good laxative.... Several swollen friends are going to plant some.... (They) are desperate and glad to hear about it."

Instant Relief for Kidney, Bladder and Urinary Problems!

Mr. H.M. writes: "Four weeks ago I developed unimaginable pain in the urinary tract which was both frightening and embarrassing. After hours of indecision I visited an emergency clinic at a very fine New York hospital, and was prescribed a sulfa drug, and was shoved out the door. Total cost: $45. Four days later the pain was worse, and swelling had spread to the prostate gland and the testicles. I went to my own doctor who gave me the choice of staying on the drug or experimenting with other drugs. I chose the new prescription.... Total cost second visit: $25.

"I tore up the prescription on the way home. By chance ...my eyes ran across an old copy of (a book of herbal remedies) ...including goldenseal, chaparral, lemon grass and Spanish eucalyptus. I purchased the teas and drank more than a quart an hour, rotating the varieties to avoid boredom. I also used a little honey. Within six hours I could urinate without pain; in the morning *all* swelling was gone from each area. I continued for three days as a safeguard.... If this can help someone in pain, I will be very happy. Total cost of teas: $6—and only a small amount of the packages were used."

Asparagus Is A Wonder Food!

Asparagus contains a large amount of a therapeutically active substance called *asparagin,* which is reportedly of great benefit in cases of kidney dysfunction. It has been said that the juice of this vegetable helps the breaking up of oxalic acid crystals in the kidneys and throughout the muscular system, and is good for rheumatism and neuritis.

Reported Cases:
- **One woman reports that asparagus therapy cured her kidney disease, which started in 1949. She had over 30 operations for kidney stones and was receiving government disability payments for "a terminal kidney condition—inoperable." She attributes the cure of this kidney trouble entirely to the asparagus therapy.**
- **A 68-year-old businessman had suffered from bladder trouble for sixteen years. After years of medical treatments, including cobalt radiation, without improvement, he went on asparagus. Within three months hospital examinations revealed that his bladder tumor had disappeared and that his kidneys were normal. Today he seems as healthy as before the disease started.**

A biochemist who studied these cases says: "I was not surprised at (these results), as a book, *The Elements of Materia Medica,* edited in 1854 by a professor at the University of Pennsylvania, states that asparagus was used as a popular remedy for kidney stones. He even refers to experiments made in 1739 on the power of asparagus to dissolve urinary stones.... Asparagus contains a good supply of proteins called 'histones' which are believed to be active in controlling cell growth ... (and) acts as a general body tonic."

This biochemist recommends cooked asparagus, blended or pureed, four tablespoons twice daily, morning and evening (diluted with water, if desired, and used as a cold or hot drink). Used this way, he says, it is a harmless substance.

Parsley—The Miracle Herb!

Parsley juice has been found valuable in removing poisons from the body. It is used medicinally for a variety of illnesses but more particularly for gravel and kidney stones, and other urinary disorders. Culpepper wrote: "The seed is effectual to break the (kidney) stones and ease the pains and torments thereof..."

Reported Cases:
- Mrs. M.D.R. reports: "I was incapacitated by what was diagnosed as toxic poisoning accompanied by a tough case of pyelitis (inflammation of the kidneys). For two years I helped support a general practitioner and a neurologist. At the end of that time I could not walk across the room without help, I had lost 50 pounds, and my pocketbook was a mere shadow of its former self.... An acquaintance asked me if I had tried parsley tea... As I had never done this, he gave me these instructions 'Take a fresh bunch of parsley... wash it in cold water. Place in a dish and cover with scalding hot water. Cover to keep warm. When cold, pour off the liquid, and drink during a 24-hour period. Repeat daily until cured.'
- "I've recommended this to many people. They never fail to get a cure, regardless of whether it is a kidney or bladder complaint. I've never known it to require more than three weeks for a cure, and have known several cases where only three days were necessary. My own case required between two and three weeks for a cure, and there has been a lapse of 35 years without a recurrence.
- "A few months ago, I heard that a friend was having kidney trouble. Without further investigation I sent her the above instructions. About a month later I received a two-page letter stating that she had been under a doctor's care for six months with two hospital confinements. She received my letter on the day that she returned from the last hospital trip, and was ready to try anything once. In three days, her urine was perfectly clear, and she was ready to resume her household duties in her mobile home. In a week's time, she was covering the park to catch up on her social obligations and tell the world about her wonderful cure."

Kidney and Prostate Relieved!

Mr. A.O. reports: "I found relief from prostate trouble —which woke me up several times nightly—with zinc gluconate. I'm free of this problem as long as I take zinc!" (It is available at most health food stores.)

"In addition, I had a very painful kidney stone that x-rays showed to be the size of a plum seed. The doctor said I could lose my kidney. I began taking 50 mg. of vitamin B-6 and magnesium oxide, 415 mg. twice daily—and found I could get relief!

"But when I ran out of zinc (for the prostate) the severe pain in my kidney returned. I am now taking 15 mg. of zinc twice daily and am happy to report my pain is gone. Needless to say, I will not be without my zinc, B-6 and magnesium."

Corn Silk Tea Soothes The Bladder!

Reportedly, corn silk tea has a smooth effect on kidney, bladder and urinary problems, and can clear up pus, infection, burning or scalding urine. It will also soothe inflammation of the urinary passages due to gravel or kidney stones, and regulate the flow of urine (whether too much or too little), in cases of bladder drip and incontinence—inability of the bladder to hold urine—and urine retention or stoppage of urine. It seems to heal diseased areas of the kidney, bladder and urinary passages and flush out uric acid, toxins and other poisons.

Reported Cases:
- **J.D. writes: "I experienced the most excruciating pain I ever felt in the form of sudden attacks of burning and scalding urine. The burning and scalding came upon me in uncontrollable waves of pain. I noticed a thick white pus dribbling out of me that turned the water a cloudy color. The flaming hot pain lasted nearly an hour. Attacks came without warning, and were especial-**

ly loathesome miles away from home. A doctor gave me a sulfa drug. This did nothing for my immediate pain and gave me nausea. Another antibiotic turned my urine red. After endless trips to the doctor, and pain so bad I nearly passed out, I tried corn silk tea. It cleared up immediately, like magic!"

- Mrs. M.B. writes: "Some years back (I am now 83) ... there seemed to be something dreadfully wrong with my kidneys. Three doctors, having taken an X-ray which showed the lower half of one kidney completely black, decided there must be an operation, at least exploratory. Deciding not to have the operation, I took my family to the country, bag and baggage, and drank corn silk tea instead of water for a year. Upon my return to the city, one of the doctors called upon me and asked, 'How are you?' I answered, 'Just fine! And you are going to laugh when I tell you I have been drinking corn silk tea.' He said, 'Well, that is nothing to laugh at—this is where they get their kidney medicine.' Another X-ray showed an entirely clean kidney. Now I swear by corn silk tea ... a proven remedy."

Mrs. M.B. adds: "Corn silks can be stored in glass jars; no need to refrigerate. One puts a handful of dried brown silks in a stew pan of water, boils it for 15 minutes to be sure it is sterile, and then drinks. It is as simple as that—no recipe is needed. It works wonders in clearing up kidney trouble." Note: corn silk may be purchased from Indiana Botanic Gardens, Hammond, Indiana 46325.

Cherry Juice for Constant Urination

Ms. J.C. writes: "I just must tell you of my discovery in hopes that someone else will find it helpful. For about five years (since age 50) I've been suffering from bladder trouble. I tried various things. ... I even went to a medical doctor who claimed I needed hormones. ... But nothing really helped. I was getting up from one to five times a night and urinating every hour or so during the day. This was most inconvenient to say the least....

> "I found help in a most unexpected way. Six months ago ... in the refrigerator I found a bottle of cherry juice. I drank it up during the course of a week, just to keep it from spoiling. I wasn't expecting anything to happen, so imagine my surprise when I realized my bladder trouble was better....

"I've continued to improve and improve. In fact, I have just slept seven hours without getting up.... I scarcely know I have a bladder any more—no more tripping to the rest room every hour on the hour. How much cherry juice wrought this miracle? I get the concentrate from the health food store, of course, and use one tablespoon in a glass of water each morning. That's it. I hope that others will find relief from this simple remedy."

Cherry Juice For Urinary Pain!

Ms. S.A. reports: "For eighteen years, I had a urinary problem—even going to the hospital at times for a 'stretching' so that I could void properly—and then within a week I'd be back in the same situation—each trip to the doctor costing $65. Finally I heard about cherry juice. I had little faith in it, but feeling that I would lose nothing by trying it (black cherry juice), and lo and behold, it works. Words can't express the wonderful feeling it is to be able to void normally—without pain."

Immediate Relief for Bladder Infection!

Mrs. E.L. writes: "It is just a year since I last took any medication for bladder infection and a year since I've been free from it. This is after more than 40 years of this scourge! Nothing ever really helped for long. Canned cranberry juice did nothing.

> "This is what helped. I ground up fresh cranberries in the food chopper. Even half a case may see you through the year. Mix with this enough unheated honey to make it palatable. Put away in cartons. At the first indication of trouble, I started eating it. With plain yogurt it is a delicious, satisfying bed-time snack.

"During the last full siege I had, the kind that hits within an hour, symptoms were greatly relieved in six hours and completely gone in 12—no medications! Now I can take warning from a slight change in the odor of the urine and start eating cranberries."

Garlic and Cystitis!

Urinary infections can be painful and debilitating. Mrs. N.Q. tells how garlic was used to relieve a persistent bladder infection:

> "For those of you who may be suffering from cystitis, garlic may be the answer. After having it several times, I decided to try my own remedy. I chopped up three large cloves of garlic three times a day, put them on a teaspoon and into my mouth and washed them down with water. After five days, the cystitis was gone. So easy ...

"I've had cystitis once since then and the garlic worked again. Maybe it will work for kidney infections, too. My doctor wasn't all too surprised as she once had a patient with lung cancer that lived longer than she expected him to and he ate garlic. The wonder drug—it really works!"

Garlic and Bladder Incontinence!

Reportedly, a woman was suffering from high blood pressure and bladder incontinence, and both were apparently relieved with a remedy involving garlic. In his book, *Of Men and Plants*, Maurice Mességué gives a remedy for bladder incontinence (inability of the bladder to hold urine), as follows:

Garlic (one large crushed head)
Single-seed hawthorn (blossoms—one handful)
Buttercup (leaves and flowers—one handful)

It is prepared, following the basic instructions on page 37 of Chapter 2, and applied to the body by sponging it on in the form of hip baths. *This mixture is not to be eaten or taken internally.*[1]

In the case of this woman, Marian O., after just a few short days of application, she reported great relief. Here was a woman of 55 who had suffered for years from incontinence —frequent urination—and bladder trouble. The constant dripping and wetness had caused her much embarrassment over the years. Her social life was at a standstill—she almost never left the house. Her blood pressure was rather high, and she complained of throbbing headaches, weakness, dizziness and fatigue.

The hip baths[2] seemed to work miracles for her. She reported much less dripping and frequency of urination, and for the first time in a long while she was able to get a good night's sleep without constantly having to run to the bathroom. Her headaches faded away and her blood pressure dropped to normal.

Massage: Miracle Medicine
Food For Your Kidneys!

Massaging the bottom of each foot at the center, or the center of each hand, with a pressure or rolling motion, may bring dramatic relief from kidney problems. If tender, do it only a few moments at a time, several times a day. Also

---

[1] Reprinted with permission of Macmillan Publishing Co., Inc., from *Of Men and Plants* by Maurice Mességué. Copyright © 1972 by Weidenfeld & Nicolson Ltd. Copyright © 1973 by Macmillan Publishing Co., Inc.,

[2] J.F. Dastur, in his book *Medicinal Plants of India*, recommends that a garlic poultice be applied to the pubic region, as well as the abdomen, in cases of urine *retention* due to atony of the bladder.

massage the bladder nerves—a little past the center on the inner edge of each foot toward the heel, to relieve stones. It may also help to massage the center of each wrist, near the palm. One man who did this, Mr. R.A., says: "In about ten minutes, I went to the bathroom and passed a stone... big enough to make a big splash when it hit the water."

A Miraculous Cure For Kidney Disease!

Kidney stone pain has been described as the most excruciating pain the body can endure, with sudden grating pain in the back, side and legs that won't go away. Sufferers may not drink enough water. *The British Medical Journal*, February 13, 1965, says that among those who drank large amounts of water (three to four quarts daily), "clear signs of stone dissolution have appeared, results sometimes being spectacular." No cure claimed.

Lack of magnesium oxide may cause kidney stones. Loring S., 33, had been passing a kidney stone every two weeks for years. Nothing he tried could stop it. Then his doctor recommended 420 mg. of magnesium-oxide tablets daily. He soon stopped passing stones and remained free of them!

One expert says that mind-power is 100 percent effective in curing kidney disease, and can restore the victim to perfect health. Miss T.R. was dying of a rare kidney disease. Several friends got together and concentrated around the clock for a month, visualizing her completely cured. At the end of that time she experienced an instantaneous healing, and felt like a new woman. Tests showed no more disease. It was miracle medicine food for her!

6

Miracle Medicine Foods For Diabetics!

Fact: the use of garlic had reduced blood sugar in diabetes. In one case, Ted V., a man with advanced diabetes, was told by doctors his condition was hopeless, and was sent home to die at age 60.

At age 90, he was still alive, in excellent health! He had started eating a combination of garlic, parsley and watercress! His blood sugar dropped from over 200 to 110! And he went on happily using this remedy for many, many years!

This is not to say that every diabetic should switch to garlic. Diabetes is such a complicated ailment that *no diabetic should ever make a single move without first securing his doctor's permission*.

It is a startling and interesting fact, however, which has been recorded several times—with the use of garlic alone. Here are some more reported cases of garlic in diabetes.

Some More Startling Facts!

The use of garlic reduced the blood sugar in a case of diabetes reported by Dr. Madaus in the German publication *Lehrbuch der Biologischen Heilmittle*, volume 1, page 479. In the December 29, 1973 issue of *Lancet*, the British medical journal, two Indian doctors point out that garlic—though a little slower in action—is as effective as tolbutamide (an oral drug for diabetics) in clearing the bloodstream of excess glucose.

Miss S.L., a garlic user, reports: "Recently, I was diagnosed as having mild diabetes. The doctor told me I would have to take an oral drug if my blood sugar didn't drop. I had read how garlic can lower blood sugar. So I immediately began taking a five-grain garlic capsule along with my vitamins and brewer's yeast after each meal. The result—my blood sugar fell to normal and no drug was needed or prescribed!"

What Is Diabetes?

There are several types of diabetes, the most common of which is *diabetes mellitus*. This is a disease which has been recognized since antiquity. A Greek by the name of Aretaeus named the disorder diabetes because it means "to run through a siphon," which refers to the great volume of urine formed in this condition. In 1675, the urine was described as being characteristically sweet. Thus the disease became known as diabetes mellitus: *mellitus* means "sweet."

In diabetes, the pancreas does not produce enough insulin —a hormone which makes it possible for sugar to enter the cells to be converted into energy. When the pancreas malfunctions, sugar can neither enter the cells nor be stored as body fat. Sugar coming from digested foods therefore accumulates in the blood until it spills over into the urine.

Insulin, given to a person with diabetes, causes the sugar to pass into the cells. In this manner, such a person can live a relatively normal life for years—as long as he gets his insulin injections (or other drugs that stimulate sugar metabolism, with all their possible side effects).

If he doesn't get his drugs, the cells of his body become starved for sugar. Symptoms such as weakness, dizziness, cold sweats, excessive thirst, and frequent urination occur—ultimately leading to blackout, shock and death. (Actually, this is an oversimplification, because the diabetic may develop kidney trouble, high blood pressure, heart failure, and a host of other symptoms.)

The Importance of Following
A Physician's Advice

It is important to know these things—to be on the alert—for the sake of *early* detection and diagnosis, which can only be done by a doctor.

That is because in early, or light cases of diabetes the sufferer need not be chained to a hypodermic needle for the rest of his or her life! Methods of treatment other than insulin are available—provided your doctor approves.

Once insulin treatment has begun, it cannot be stopped. It must be used religiously, for the rest of the patient's life, because—in most cases—the pancreas then *stops* producing what little insulin it can. There is virtually no hope of healing. It means *daily injections,* because insulin cannot be swallowed (the stomach digests or neutralizes insulin).

That is why doctors explore every possibility—such as the use of orinase, a milder drug in tablet form, or simply a special drug-free diet (low on foods that overwork the pancreas)—before prescribing insulin. *All these measures and more can work in early or light cases,* because carbohydrate (sugar) metabolism is not influenced solely by insulin. A host of other glands and organs, such as the adrenals, secretes hormones which are vitally important in the regulation of blood sugar.

Garlic contains certain minerals of proven value in carbohydrate metabolism. It is not the only food which contains them, but it may be a very rich source, in view of the fact that it has helped control diabetes in actual, documented cases. Discuss it with your doctor.

Possible Effect Of Garlic
On Diabetes

Garlic is rich in potassium (529 mg. in 100 grams). In diabetes, excess acidity (acidosis) can rob the body of so much potassium that unconsciousness or diabetic coma can result. As one authority puts it:

> "Diabetic patients are frequently deficient in potassium, which, though needed to utilize sugar, drops far below normal when the blood sugar falls or acidosis develops."

Potassium is of proven worth in case of *low* blood sugar —which is remarkably similar to diabetes. Low blood sugar causes much potassium to be lost in the urine. Its symptoms are weakness, dizziness, headaches, trembling, sweating, and even blackout. If a normal person goes without a meal, or a diabetic takes insulin and then skips a meal, these symptoms can occur. In cases of low blood sugar, taking potassium chloride brought almost immediate relief and prevented blackouts.[1]

Possible Effects Of Other Minerals In Garlic

Garlic contains zinc—which is found in concentrated form in the liver, spleen, and *pancreas*. Zinc is a component of the insulin that diabetics take (generally "protomine zinc insulin"). It has been found that when insulin is given by injection, the addition of zinc to it prolongs its effect—spreads the insulin out in the bloodstream as slowly as possible, and makes it last longer, so that fewer injections are needed during

---

[1] In low blood sugar, the body produces too much insulin. When sugar or starch are eaten, too much insulin—secreted by the pancreas—removes them so quickly from the blood for fat storage that blood sugar level becomes extremely low, and low energy, fatigue, and headache results. The remedy for this, doctors say, is to avoid starchy, sugary foods and the fast food items (candy, chocolate, soda, pie) that low blood sugar victims often eat for a quick energy boost. These simply cause too much insulin to be produced—sugar is removed even faster—and symptoms become worse. In general, a high protein and low or natural carbohydrate (fresh fruits and vegetables) diet is recommended. Weight loss, restored energy and relief of symptoms automatically follows in most cases.

the day. According to recent research, the zinc content of the pancreas of diabetic patients is only half that of normal persons.

In his book *Nutrition and the Soil*, Picton tells us that "the medical profession as a result of investigation suggests that lack of zinc may be closely related to the onset of diabetes."

Garlic contains manganese—a trace mineral needed by humans in microscopic amounts. There is evidence that maganese is needed by diabetics. G.J. Everson and R.E. Sharder report in the *Journal of Nutrition* (94, 89, 1968) that a lack of manganese can actually affect glucose tolerance, the ability to remove excess sugar from the blood. A year earlier (*Journal of Nutrition*, 91, 453, 1967) they reported that manganese-deficient animals frequently produced offspring with pancreatic abnormalities or without a pancreas.

In humans, a manganese deficiency may contribute to diabetes. L.G. Kosenko reports (*Clinical Medicine*, 42, 113, 1964) that when 122 diabetics, ranging in age from 15 to 81, were examined, the manganese content of the blood was one-half that of normal people. The longer a patient had diabetes, the lower his manganese blood level was. In many countries, according to *Nutrition Reviews* (July 1968), plant extracts which are good sources of manganese have been used as home remedies in diabetes... such as blueberry, onion, brewer's yeast, and of course, garlic.

Finally, the mineral which gives garlic its smell—sulfur—is found in pancreatic insulin.

A Vitamin In Garlic That Acts Like Insulin!

Garlic contains vitamin C, and increases its absorption from other foods. Vitamin C acts like insulin (the hormone secreted by the pancreas), according to Professor S. Bamerjee of the School of Tropical Medicine, Calcutta, India. According to Professor Bamerjee, vitamin C—like insulin—helps metabolize carbohydrates in foods. He has also found that laboratory animals lack insulin in their systems when denied vitamin C.

Honey and Diabetes!

Honey is largely a combination of various sugars, and contains a rare type of sugar known as levulose, which has the advantage of being absorbed so slowly that it does not have the "shock" effect of other sugars, which are difficult for people with high or low blood sugar to handle. One medical doctor, an expert on honey therapy, suggests there is more than a possibility of using honey for these sufferers.

> **Another medical doctor states: "... the employment of honey in the treatment of diabetics may look antiscientific, antimedical, even rather silly to the theoretical mind, to the uninitiated, or to a superficial observer. Just at this writing, my bee flock ... is busy gathering honey from a plant now in bloom here.... We make tincture and fluid extract of this plant ... and I give it to diabetic patients in drop doses (with decidedly good effect)."**

If the plant is good for his patients, he reasons, why not the honey derived from it? Dr. A.Y. Davidov of Russia has found honey a good substitute for sugar in diabetes. One of his patients used one pound of honey in ten days without an increase of sugar in the urine. When the honey was stopped, the sugar rose. With four teaspoons of honey daily, the sugar rate dropped. He reported six more instances where honey had a beneficial effect in diabetes. Dr. L.R. Emerick of Eaton, Ohio, a specialist, used honey in the diet of more than 250 diabetic patients with success.

Seemingly Hopeless Cases Cured!

Some people claim that honey has been used by them in hopeless diabetic conditions with the best success and resulted in cures. One man writes:

- "I became a diabetic, and had to retire because I felt so weak. Doctors said there was no cure. Then I began a diet of raw vegetables sweetened with honey and lime:

spinach, lettuce, cabbage, carrots, fresh tomatoes and whole wheat bread. I began this diet around 1920, and a year later the doctors could not find a trace of sugar. Now, at 70, I can eat anything on the table, and do more work than any man my age!"

- Another man writes that he cured many cases of rheumatism and people who were diabetics with honey. He cites the case of a man and his wife who both suffered from diabetes, doctoring with various physicians for a long time without improving. Finally they went on a diet consisting of large amounts of honey and plenty of fruit, and today both are fit as a fiddle!

If you are suffering from diabetes, however, you are cautioned not to use honey without the advice and strict control of your physician.

How Diabetes Was Permanently Cured!

Around the turn of the century, Dr. Ramm, of Preetz, Germany, experimenting with the kidney bean pods, found that in diabetics, traces of sugar vanished from the urine when they drank the water in which kidney bean pods had been cooked. (See instructions in Chapter 5.) The length of time involved was three to four weeks, during which a strict diabetic diet was advised. Years before insulin, many seemingly hopeless cases were permanently cured!

Dr. Ramm reported cases of diabetics who had taken the treatment 12 years previously, were cured and stopped drinking the water—and yet had no sign of a return of the disease.

Others who did experience a return of sugar in the urine were able to find relief again by drinking the bean water for a few weeks. As with all remedies in this book, a doctor's permission is required before self-medication may be tried.

Parsley and Diabetes!

Mr. C.D. suffered from prostate enlargement, with infection and pus—and finally complete stoppage of urine. He was extremely frightened, and had fever and chills. He was rushed to a hospital, where a doctor quickly inserted a tube to drain his bladder. He could not urinate without the tube. He was told he needed surgery, but they could not operate, since he had diabetes. He was advised to try parsley tea. After drinking this tea, he could urinate freely without a tube, his sugar dropped to normal, and surgery was happily avoided! Many others report similar relief!

Blueberry Tea For High Blood Sugar!

Miss C.O. reports: "Although I was told in the hospital in March that I had a mild case of diabetes, I was determined that I would cure myself if I possibly could. I watched my eating very carefully—ate no food with sugar on or in it, used plenty of vegetables, fruits and, of course, some meat. I also took vitamins and minerals, such as bone meal, dolomite and A and D, vitamin B complex which had B-6 in it, vitamin E, vitamin C, and especially important, I used blueberry leaf tea two and three times a day. Last August 23 the doctor took my blood test; the following day he reported to me that my blood was perfectly normal, so I have no more diabetes."

Brewer's Yeast and Diabetes!

Mrs. F.M. reports: "About 2 years ago after an examination by a doctor, I discovered I had diabetes. Not bad enough yet for insulin injections. Meanwhile, I moved to another state and had another examination by another doctor. This time I was told I had no diabetes. I never knew what had brought about the cure until I read that brewer's yeast can help the pancreas produce insulin, thus helping to prevent diabetes. I have been eating brewer's yeast about a year. My favorite breakfast consists of a sliced banana covered with wheat germ, ground sunflower seeds, and brewer's yeast with milk."

100% Cure Rate Reported With Revolutionary New Diet and Exercise Program For Diabetics

Recently, a national newspaper reported that U.S. government doctors, working with 20 diabetics with average blood sugar counts of 170, obtained a 100 percent cure rate in three weeks, with a revolutionary new diet and exercise program!

The doctors at the VA Hospital in Lexington, Kentucky report that in another group, 75 percent of chronic adult diabetics—some using as much as 20 units of insulin a day—were totally off drugs, and completely symptom-free in only three weeks! Their average blood sugar count dropped from 230 to 120, normal!

A spokesman stated that on the basis of these tests, an estimated 2.5 million adult diabetics—nearly three out of four—can be controlled without drugs with this diet in as little as three weeks! The diet consists of high-carbohydrate, low-calorie foods with plenty of fiber. In addition, patients must walk a normal speed for 30 minutes, three times a day, preferably after meals. The doctors insisted that responding patients can live completely normal lives without drugs as long as they stick with the program.

Diabetic Saved From Amputation!

Mrs. S.R., a diabetic, was suffering from a horrible infection in her foot. She was in excruciating pain, and could hardly walk. Doctors had removed one toe, and wanted to amputate her entire foot.

Then she heard how diabetics can avoid amputation due to early hardening of the arteries and bad circulation in

the legs by soaking them in warm (not hot) salt water, or peroxide and water.

This she did, and a week later her doctor was amazed! It was almost completely healed! No amputation needed, as X-rays proved. Pain and swelling were gone, and she was pronounced cured! For Mrs. S.R. warm salt-water foot baths were miracle medicine food, as her doctor observed!

Vitamin E Healed Gangrene!

In "Alphatocopherol in the Management of Small Areas of Gangrene" (*Canadian Medical Association Journal*, May 1, 1957), Drs. Stephen Tolgys and Evan Shute say that about 50 percent of patients with gangrene, resulting from arteriosclerosis, diabetes and Buerger's disease, were saved from amputation by vitamin E. A 30-year-old man had gangrene patches on the fingers of one hand. Using 500 mg. of vitamin E and nothing else except vitamin E ointment, it healed completely in two months. Observers state that it was "hard to believe that the hideous purple and black patches" could be changed to "normal pink tissue with no other treatment than this miracle medicine food, vitamin E.

7

Miracle Medicine Foods For The Stomach!

Indigestion! All of us experience it at one time or another—heaviness after eating, gas, belching, nausea, and often heart palpitations and severe headaches. Commercial alkalizers work, but they deplete the stomach's supply of hydrochloric acid, without which food is not fully digested. Actual vitamin and mineral deficiencies can—and do—develop.

What can be done to relieve this situation—quickly, easily, and conveniently—without the use of chemical drugs? First, a diet emphasizing natural foods—garlic foods, lean meat, fish, poultry, fresh vegetables and fruits —will do wonders to maintain a healthful acid/alkaline balance in the stomach.

Anything that produces excess acid (sugars, starches, pastries, smoking) may be reduced or eliminated with wonderful results. In a natural, drugless way, nature can bring instant relief for stomach and intestines.

Nature's Own "Magic Pink Pill"

Papaya is a peach-like tropical fruit, valued for its powerful digestive enzyme called *papain*. Most health food stores sell papaya in convenient sliced and bottled form. The enzyme is also available in delicious chewable tablets at health stores everywhere. Papaya has proved invaluable in cases of feeble digestion, gas, heartburn, diarrhea, and the incomplete digestion of foods known as drop syndrome. It is especially valuable for those who have trouble digesting meat, eggs and protein. It is so powerful, its extract is used as a *meat tenderizer!*

> **J.P., an 80-year-old man who ran a rooming house, had to greet guests hobbling painfully on crutches. He could not digest anything, until someone told him about papaya. He started eating this miracle medicine food and gained strength. Soon he put aside his crutches and was so active he ran errands in his spare time to stores in the city 2 miles away!**

For five years, Gloria T. had a large growth in her abdomen, too big to remove surgically. It was very painful. Doctors were not sure of its cause, even after an exploratory operation. Finally, her doctor advised her to try a mango-and-papaya diet. The hard mass in her stomach and intestines began to disappear, until finally the entire area was soft, and appeared normal, without pain.

Enzyme Tablets Are Miracle Medicine Food!

Mr. E.R. reports: "Five years ago I was operated on for ulcers, and ¾ of my stomach was removed. After the operation, I never felt the same. I was always bloated after eating, with gas in stomach and intestines which drove me back and forth to doctors, but all I got was tranquilizers of all sorts. They claimed it was my nerves. My diet was restricted to all bland foods. Even with pills and special food, my diarrhea was bad. With loose bowels on and off since my operation, I lost weight. Seems I developed a drop syndrome. Food went in and out within a half hour.

> **"I'm not a doctor, but I believed because I had no stomach, that food went into my bowels not fully digested and the work load was all in the intestines. Food not**

fully digested was expelled almost as eaten. One day I saw an ad about enzyme tablets. I tried everything else, so why not one more? Believe me, I never thought there would be an improvement.

"Enzymes aid in digestion. My gas pains practically disappeared! I feel 100 percent better. I wish my doctor had told me about this aid to digestion. I would not have suffered five years needlessly."

Bleeding Ulcers Disappear—Surgery Avoided!

In one reported case, Mr. R.Y., 25 suffered bleeding ulcers. He had been in and out of hospitals every week for over a year—once for a three week stay—and doctors were urging the removal of a portion of his stomach. He was about ready for that—anything to relieve his terrible pain.

Instead, he decided to take his mother's advice and agreed to eat only what she gave him: health foods, sprouts, juices, eggs, cottage cheese, home-baked breads, brewer's yeast, desiccated liver, wheat germ, fortified milk (every five hours for the first two weeks) and maximum doses of every vitamin, including 30 mg. of zinc per day.

"Within two months," it is reported, "he had no ulcers, and his general health improved vastly." He forgot all about his ulcer medicine!

Heartburn and Ulcers Relieved Instantly!

Cabbage contains the anti-ulcer vitamin, U, plus chlorine and sulfur which helps cleanse the mucous membranes of the stomach. This, say medical authorities, is only possible if eaten *raw* or its fresh juice drunk. The value of raw cabbage juice as a cure for ulcers is now recognized by many doctors, since it was first announced by Dr. Garnett Cheney of the Department of Medicine, Stanford University Medical School, around 1950.

Mr. L.W. reports: "I was at home feeling punk and feeling sorry for myself. I had just gotten word from my physician that x-rays showed my old ulcer had returned, and on top of that I had a new one. Once again, I was faced with the healing up of two of the pesky things with the old antacid treatment. Then I heard about cabbage for ulcers. So I brought out my old vegetable juicer. I started with five glasses of cabbage juice the first day and almost at once, there was no pain. I continued this for another week, and then reduced it to three glasses per day. Both ulcers were healed when I had my check-up x-rays two months later. I am sure they were healed several weeks before the check-up because I had no pain or discomfort. I thought you might like to know it really works."

If I may interject a personal opinion here, I do not believe the healing occurred on account of so-called "vitamin U," a hypothetical substance about which very little is known. I believe it was simply due to the vitamin C content of cabbage. However little they received of it, vitamin C or ascorbic acid is something which ulcer patients are usually denied. Doctors often believe it irritates the stomach. But how can the tissue breakdown—which is what an ulcer is— heal without vitamin C, the main ingredient of collagen (tissue cement)? Just as the modest C content of cabbage was enough to prevent scurvy, during the early sea voyages, I believe it simply healed the ulcers in these patients, as well.

Reported Cases:
- Jordan H., 52, was suffering from an acute peptic ulcer. He needed surgery but had to wait for a hospital bed. In order to give him immediate relief, his doctor suggested a quart of fresh cabbage juice (four glasses) a day. In a matter of days, he was feeling fine, and cancelled his surgery!
- A man, diagnosed at a famous clinic as suffering from a brain tumor and a stomach ulcer, was told by his doctor to take four glasses of raw cabbage juice a day, stop smoking, and eat natural foods. In a short time, his ulcer vanished. Even more amazing, the brain tumor disappeared and he was completely normal!

A Cure for Acid Indigestion (Diverticulitis Relieved)!

Mrs. O.C. reports: "My husband has discovered a simple and effective cure for acid indigestion. I have diverticulitis so I was bothered quite a bit, especially every night, with upset stomach and acid rising into my throat, whereupon I'd take commercial alkalizers for relief. One night my husband also had acid indigestion and he ate a *radish* and that was it! One large radish acts like magic, instantly quieting all symptoms of indigestion!"

Can Garlic Cure Stomach Aliments?

Taken regularly, garlic can cure stomach and intestinal ailments, says a leading scientist and expert on garlic therapy. Reportedly, the allicin in garlic stimulates the walls of the stomach and intestines to secrete digestive enzymes. But garlic taken by people suffering from such conditions must be diluted or mixed with other foods, says this expert. An excellent way to tame garlic is to cook it, or mix it with egg and milk.

Garlic need not even be eaten, however. Externally, garlic may be used in poultices or foot- and hand-baths to soothe the stomach. Used in this manner it has been reported 95 percent effective.

Praised The World Over!

From ancient times to the present, garlic has been praised the world over for relief of gas, cramps and catarrhal (inflammation) symptoms. The classic work in this area that finally established a firm scientific basis for use of garlic in stomach and digestive disorders, was done by Damrau and Ferguson, and reported in the *Review of Gastroenterology* for May 1949. Fifty-four patients were treated. Each was given two garlic tablets twice daily, after lunch and dinner, for a period of two weeks.

All Symptoms Relieved!

Wonderful results were reported, which were tabulated and reported in full detail as follows:

- Heaviness after eating was completely relieved in 15 cases, and partially relieved in six out of 25—for a total of 84 percent effectiveness!
- Belching was completely relieved in 13 cases, partially in nine—out of 25—a total of 88 percent effectiveness!
- Flatulence was completely relieved in 20 cases out of 25—a total of 80 percent effectiveness!
- Gas colic was completely relieved in 13 cases, and partially relieved in eight—a total of 84 percent effectiveness!
- Nausea was completely relieved in six out of eight cases —for a total of 75 percent effectiveness!

It is reported that garlic brought not just temporary relief, but permanent freedom from these gastric disorders. The researchers concluded that garlic is a carminative which may be used in flatulence and colic, to expel gas from stomach and intestines and to diminish the gripping pains.

How Garlic May Be Used To Soothe Stomach and Digestion!

Externally, garlic may be used in poultices or foot- and hand-baths (see Chapter 2 and 4). Internally, diced garlic may be taken with honey, before or after meals (use half a clove). Garlic may also be used in the form of garlic tablets or capsules; follow label instructions. These are available without prescription at health food stores. They have the advantage of being tasteless and odorless, for those who shy away from garlic in the raw.

Garlic Claimed 95% Effective In Digestive Disorders!

In his book, *Of Men and Plants,* Maurice Mességué reports 95 percent effectiveness (80 percent cured, 15 percent greatly relieved) in cases of digestive disorders, with the following remedy—a prime ingredient of which is garlic—

for use as an abdominal poultice, and in hand-baths, only: it is not to be taken internally.[1]

DISORDERS OF THE DIGESTION
Garlic (one large crushed head)
Roman chamomile (one dozen crushed heads)
Peppermint (leaves—one handful)
Thyme (leaves—one handful)

Follow the directions for making a poultice on page 78, Chapter 4, using nettle (fresh leaves if possible) and watercress (one bunch, chopped). The basic preparation should be made by following the directions on page 37, Chapter 2. Pour a liqueur glass full of the basic preparation over the poultice. This should be applied hot, after meals, says Mességué. Hand baths may be prepared with the basic preparation only.

Mességué gives two other external applications using garlic for use in cases of stomach upset:[2]

DYSPEPSIA
Garlic (one large crushed head)
Milfoil (flowers—one handful)
Cow-parsnip (root, leaves, seed—one handful, mixed)
Roman chamomile (one dozen crushed heads) *or*
Peppermint (leaves—one handful)
Yellow gentian (root—one large pinch)
Round-leaved mallow (leaves and flowers—one handful)
Thyme (leaves—one handful)

Use in foot and hand baths.

---

[1] Reprinted with permission of Macmillan Publishing Co., Inc., from *Of Men and Plants* by Maurice Mességué. Copyright © 1972 by Weidenfeld & Nicolson Ltd. Copyright © 1973 by Macmillan Publishing Co., Inc.,
[2] *Of Men and Plants* by Maurice Mességué, *Ibid.*

GASTRALGIA

>Garlic (one crushed head)
>Milfoil (flowers—one handful)
>Single seed hawthorn (blossom—one handful)
>Corn poppy (flowers and capsules—one handful)
>Round-leaved mallow (flowers and leaves—one handful)
>Blackberry bramble (leaves—one handful)

Hot compresses to be applied to the stomach. Hand baths.

Remarkable Results!

In the *Review of Gastroenterology* for January-February 1944 Harry Barowsky and Linn J. Boyd, both physicians, tell of using garlic on fifty patients who suffered from "various disorders commonly associated with gastrointestinal symptoms." Flatulence (gas) was relieved in the vast majority of cases. Relief from nausea, vomiting, abdominal distention and after-meal discomfort was also reported.

In short, garlic—taken in tablet or capsule form, or as an excellent food in its own right—can be helpful in correcting many of the symptoms arising from digestive upset.

A Vitamin In Garlic That Has Healed Ulcers!

Garlic contains vitamin C, and increases its absorption from other foods with which it is eaten. Several researchers have shown that vitamin C serves as an excellent therapeutic measure in cases of ulcer. In fact, a lack of vitamin C may *cause* stomach and duodenal ulcers.

Two researchers, Eddy and Dahldorf, tell of a group of ulcer patients who were put on a bland diet, low in vitamin C. (Because vitamin C is an acid, many doctors are afraid to use it on such patients.) In 15 days, the patients began experiencing symptoms of vitamin C deficiency. Then vitamin C was added to their diet. As a result, 70 percent of these ulcer patients were cured![3]

The British Medical Journal, May 17, 1947, details a case in which the patient was hemorrhaging from the digestive tract. Because he had a peptic (stomach) ulcer, he had been advised to avoid vitamin C for several years. Within half an hour after 1000 mg. of vitamin C was given to him intravenously, the patient—who had been near death—became alert and cheerful. He stopped bringing up blood and was considered healed.

Comfrey: The Simple Country Remedy That Worked Miracles!

Comfrey is a common kitchen herb, possessing extraordinary healing powers. This is due to a substance it contains called *allantoin*. It is difficult to dismiss the old wives' tales about this herb. Read these and judge for yourself:

- In a miraculous case, Mr. Emmet T., 60, suffering pain after food, vomiting of blood, and other ulcer symptoms —with no relief from medicines—finally agreed to an operation. He nearly died on the operating table after the stomach (with an ulcer in it) had been exposed. The operation had to be abandoned, and the ulcer remained. He was then treated with allantoin dissolved in a comfrey infusion and a purely milk diet, with the result that he was completely free of ulcers in a month, and has lived to nearly 100!
- In another case, Mrs. Sylvia D., 42, was near death with a seemingly cancerous tumor on her right side. She was given a mucilaginous infusion of comfrey root reinforced with a solution of allantoin. In a month the tumor disappeared. The diagnosis was changed to nonmalignant!

---

[3] Eddy and Dahldorf, *The Avitaminoses* (Williams and Wilkins).

- Jeanne B., 16, suffered from a bleeding stomach ulcer, with nausea and vomiting. The doctor put her on the usual diet, with medication, warning her to stay away from certain foods. In a matter of days, she was completely healed—later confessing that she never took a drop of the doctor's medicine. All she did was sip strong comfrey tea until she felt healed.

Hopeless Cases Cured—With Honey!

Dr. Schacht, of Weisbaden, Germany, claims to have cured many hopeless cases of gastric and intestinal ulcers with honey, without operations. Another medical doctor states that "honey will cure gastric and intestinal ulcerations" which he calls a "distressing...and most dangerous malady, a precursor of cancer." But he says the news has not yet reached 99 percent of the medical profession, and those who *do* know it are afraid to say so for fear of being laughed at by their colleagues! Father Kneipp the great naturalist, stated: "Smaller ulcers of the stomach are quickly contracted, broken and healed by (honey)."

One man reports: "I have been a sufferer from ulcerated stomach for several years, part time in the hospital, part time in bed, and nearly all the time in much pain. I noticed (after eating honey) that I was much better and gave no thought to the reason, but kept up eating honey because I relished it. I've had no attacks since."

Powdered Okra For Ulcers and Colitis!

The thick, gooey nature of okra when cooked or used in soup makes it suitable for treatment of stomach ulcers and inflammation of the colon (colitis). It was observed by a certatin doctor that a patient who had mucous colitis, a disorder in which there are alternating attacks of constipation and diarrhea, was improved by using a large amount of okra. This led Dr. J. Meyer of Chicago and his co-workers to make a study of okra.

Seventeen persons with ulcers of the stomach or the first part of the intestines were given powdered okra as the only form of treatment for their condition. The diagnosis was made in each case by means of X-rays. Of the seventeen patients who were treated, fourteen received immediate relief of their symptoms!

According to studies by Dr. Evans and Drs. Meyer, E.E. Seidman, and H. Necheles, it was found that taking okra powder not only eased the discomfort but also caused the stomach to empty more promptly.

Okra is delicious when cooked or added to vegetable soup. For more effective medicinal purposes, it should be run through a juicer and the juice used for drinking and/or gargling for sore throat. It has also been found to be valuable for cases of inflammation of the membrane surrounding the lungs (pleurisy).

Celery For Heartburn!

Miss E.C. reports: "During my first pregnancy, I was prone to heartburn and discovered eating a stick of celery would relieve the discomfort. Celery was a must on our rides, trips or wherever we went. A bunch of celery sticks tied in a plastic bag was my remedy and a wonderful snack for other children with us. This is also a healthy way to hold down weight that becomes a problem during pregnancy!"

Ulcer Cured By Goat's Milk!

Mrs. K.M. reports: "A man in our area had ulcers and was pronounced 'incurable' by 15 doctors. An old timer told him to live on goat's milk. He tried it and, as proven by an x-ray, his ulcers have completely disappeared!"

More Miracle Medicine Foods for Your Ulcer!

Nerve massage can relieve ulcer pain, in minutes, and often brings complete cures, says experts. To relieve ulcers, massage the soft pad at the base of the thumb, near the web, on each hand. Then massage the webs (this can also relieve hiccoughs, and rubbing the little finger and the one next to it can often relieve car sickness). We are told of a woman, suffering from excruciating ulcer pain in her stomach, who was given this miracle medicine food. She felt immediate relief, sighing, "There, that hits the spot!" In less than five minutes, her pain was completely gone.

Emotional problems can hurl you into a severe case of heartburn and ulcer symptoms. Mind power can relieve these symptoms in every case, one expert going so far as to say that positive thinking can completely heal any ulcer, no matter how severe it may be. This miracle medicine food will guarantee you and your loved ones freedom from ulcers, says this expert, adding that it not only rids the body of pain, but heals the ulcer itself!

8

Miracle Medicine Foods For Constipation, Diarrhea, Colitis And Other Intestinal Ailments!

High fiber foods, including fresh fruits, nuts, vegetables, seeds, cereals with bran, and whole wheat bread, may be regarded as miracle medicine foods for constipation. Even more remarkable, studies have shown that high fiber foods can help prevent conditions such as gallstones, stomach ailments and circulatory problems, including hemorrhoids and varicose veins!

Like A Prayer Answered!

Mrs. V.E. reports: "Since losing a tremendous amount of weight (from 230 to 110) I have had trouble with my bowels. I was usually constipated and when I did go I had to strain so hard my face turned beet red. My doctor put me on a low residue diet which just seemed to make matters worse. Then I heard about unprocessed bran and wheat germ. I took one tablespoon of each in coffee twice a day, and it was like a prayer answered.

"I immediately started having normal bowel movements every morning, in which I felt for the first time I was really emptying my bowels. I now take one tablespoon of each just in the morning with my coffee with the same results. I was really surprised to find out just how many people have the same problem and now have several friends taking it too.

"What really surprises me the most is, how come doctors never recommend this as a treatment? Is it because they just don't know about bran and wheat germ, or they don't really care? When I told my own doctor he looked surprised and asked me if it *really* worked."

After Many Years, Relief With Natural Bran!

Mr. L.E. reports: "I suffered from constipation for many years, going two and three days frequently between eliminations. Many times I strained at stool and elimination was frequently a painful experience. Then I learned about the benefits of unprocessed bran. I rushed out and bought some, and have been eating a rounded teaspoon once a day, at breakfast, for a little over a year.

"**Elimination has become a pleasure—no pain, no straining. Elimination has occurred at least once a day and frequently two or three times a day. If anyone is suffering from constipation and its many symptoms and side effects, try bran and you will like it.**"

Mrs. W.V. reports: "For seven years I did not have a normal bowel movement. I went to the Wheeling Clinics and had every test there was to take. I went to doctors, who made me worse with prescriptions. I felt I was a hopeless case until a friend told me about natural bran. For 59 cents I got relief."

Reported Cases:
- Mrs. S.G. reports: "I used to be constipated all the time for years, getting relief only from enemas. Now, after eating raw fruit and taking many food supplements, I have two or three bowel movements a day."
- Mrs. N.J. writes: "I have been suffering all my life with constipation. I have tried everything anyone ever told

me but nothing worked including natural bran. Then I noticed that papaya was an aid to digestion so I tried taking it. Much to my surprise I found my problem solved.... It's worth a try and since it is so tasty and easy to take, also inexpensive, you have nothing to lose." (Papaya also comes in tasty tablet form.)

- Mr. E.D.B. writes: "I want to say that sunflower seeds wear the crown when it comes to regularity. They act as a laxative and also provide the body with much good nutrition, so they can't help but improve general health. I buy sunflower seeds in bulk and distribute them to my friends. One friend was constipated for years. Sunflower seeds were the answer for him."

Famous Remedies For Constipation!

One of the mildest laxatives is olive oil (one tablespoon at bedtime). In enema form it is often used to relieve fecal impaction or blockage. Figs have been recommended—in a one-day program of figs and nothing else. The simple addition of bananas to the diet is often helpful. Constipation is often relieved in long-standing (20-year) sufferers by the simple addition of more water to the diet. A glass of tap water *before* orange juice and cereal at breakfast, and at least one more glass of water before bedtime, is usually recommended by doctors.

Charles G., 58, was so completely constipated he thought he had a growth or polyps or some kind of intestinal blockage. An old Italian doctor said frankly, "You don't need any laxatives, or even an operation. I'll tell you what: you go home, buy some escarole (at your local supermarket—it looks like lettuce), boil it in water, and drink the water." It worked like magic!

From that moment on, he had no pain, no straining, and completely natural evacuations. A friend, Beverly F., 34, upon hearing of this, also decided to try escarole. She had become very constipated ever since having a baby years ago. But instead of boiling it and drinking the water (she didn't have time), she ate some raw, the first thing in the morning. It worked amazingly well, just like the doctor said. All of which seems to prove—the next time you're in pain, instead of going to your local druggist who'll charge you a fortune (and fill you with chemicals), try your local supermarket, where you can get relief for a few cents!

Enlarged Hemorrhoids Disappear!

Constipation often results in hemorrhoids. A good remedy for hemorrhoids is chopped green onions, mixed with wheat flour, fried in animal fat, spread on cloth and applied just before bedtime. Repeat as needed. It is said this remedy will relieve the condition in two days!

> Mr. W.N. reports: "After suffering on and off for several years I tried applying Lecithin 1200, a rather gelatinous concentration of the soybean extract. The effect was miraculous. Application was made once a day for two or three days, and the enlarged hemorrhoids completely disappeared. They have not returned. This cure happened after everything else had failed."

Mr. M.T. reports: "I was having a great deal of trouble with hemorrhoids. The swelling was bad and the pain was terrible. I tried various remedies and nothing seemed to help. Then ... I started to use rutin and got relief within just a few days. A friend of mine was having the same trouble. He also used it and got help immediately. I have continued taking rutin since that time as it is very cheap and will help prevent the hemorrhoids from returning."

Immediate Relief For Hemorrhoids!

Mrs. H.B. says: "About a month ago I had a severe intestinal virus that had me in the bathroom continually for six days. The constant diarrhea so aggravated the hemorrhoids that I developed while pregnant with my children that I was absolutely miserable. After a few days of applying vitamin E, castor oil, and a popular remedy sold over the counter, none of which brought much relief, I called a very knowledgable friend to ask her advice.

"What she told me to do brought immediate relief and is absolutely amazing! I put a small handful of cranberries in the blender to chop them finely. Then I wrap about one tablespoon or so in a piece of cheesecloth and tuck it in the area. Within 30 minutes I could feel the pain being drawn out.

"After about an hour when the cloth begins to turn color from bright red to brownish, apply a new compress. I am not exaggerating when I tell you that two hours later I felt great and slept through the entire night without waking from the pain. Although I do recognize and prefer natural remedies, I must admit that I did not really believe or understand how cranberries could help, but because I have such respect for my friend I gave it a try. You can be sure that although I almost never have this kind of problem, a bag of cranberries will be in my freezer just in case."

Pain Relieved Immediately!

Mr. N.T. writes! "For a long time I had been subject to recurring attacks (spaced several years apart) of external hemorrhoids. Commercial preparations did no good; prescriptions were no better. Generally, the attack ended with a minor operation at the doctor's office, after which there was a slow, painful recovery. Then my doctor moved away, which posed a dilemma when the next attack arrived. Having read of the marvelous results of vitamin E with burns and skin ailments, I decided to apply it—half as a suppository, half externally using a pierced 100 I.U. capsule for each treatment. The pain left almost immediately ... with complete recovery in about two weeks. Steady application and patience are required."

Unbearable Rectal Itch Completely Relieved!

Mrs. E.D. reports: "For some time I had been plagued by rectal itching. A certain commercial preparation brought only temporary relief. One day I thought of vinegar. As it turned out a wad of raw cotton thoroughly saturated in ordinary vinegar and applied overnight has brought total relief until now—many months later! If the area has been irritated through scratching there will, of course, be a temporary burning sensation. I have discovered that vinegar will also bring immediate relief and quick cure for poison oak or ivy. Apply several times a day."

Mr. B.J. reports: "I have scratched my rear end for over 15 years and have been told by doctors it was caused by antibiotics killing off the bacteria in my bowels. I have been prescribed buttermilk, yogurt and various salves to ease my discomfort. Needless to say, none has been very lasting. Then I discovered wheat germ oil!

"I just washed myself with soap, rinsed off and dried with a tissue, and then applied the wheat germ oil to all affected parts. It's been almost two weeks and I have not had even a twinge of an itch and no sores. Only someone who has scratched for as long as I have can understand the wonderful relief."

Rectal Sores Relieved!

Rectal sores *must* be examined by a qualified doctor to determine if they are harmless. If they are harmless, here is a remedy that may clear them up completely. Mrs. L.E. reports: "For over two years, I have been afflicted with sores in the anal area. In the last six months they started to get serious, particularly when I had a bowel movement. I went to all kinds of doctors and each one gave me a different drug ointment. It did not clear up and grew steadily worse. I was on my way to becoming a partial invalid because of the pain and deterioration of the entire area. Finally I was given x-ray treatments but this did not clear it up. Back again came the sores with ferocious intensity.

"In desperation, I decided to use home treatments. For the first time in two years I have cleared it up completely and it has not returned yet. The real miracle is wheat germ oil. In the morning, I use very hot water, bathing the area for two minutes, then apply wheat germ oil for two minutes. Wash lightly with a non-irritating soap, rinse again in hot water and wash it again.

"Allow to dry without touching. Drying is important. Then apply wheat germ oil and keep it applied all day. I carry capsules with me and apply one when convenient. At night I repeat the entire procedure. A bit complicated, but you will be amazed how it improves." Wheat germ contains vitamin E which healed it.

Pain Of Hemorrhoids Stopped In Minutes!

Reportedly, in hundreds of cases, hemorrhoid pain was stopped in minutes, completely and permanently, never to return again—even in severe cases—with nerve massage. One woman suffered from such painful bleeding hemorrhoids that she thought she had cancer, because they refused to heal. Yet her doctor couldn't see anything wrong. With this miracle medicine food for hemorrhoids—nerve massage—her hemorrhoids were relieved in five minutes and never bothered her again!

With this method, hemorrhoids will vanish in two or three days, says one expert. Start by massaging the bony edges of the heels of your feet, and the palms of your hands, with a press and roll motion. Then with your thumbs, massage up the center of your arms, from wrist to elbow.

Miracle Medicine Foods Relieve Ulcerative Colitis!

Ulcerative colitis is a severe form of diarrhea, at times alternating with constipation. Mrs. J.S. reports: "I am now 33 years old. I was stricken with ulcerative colitis when I was 11 years old. There were many many loopholes in what the doctors told me. Pickles and milk, etc., did not bother me. My pains were not in the 'right places,' and much to their bewilderment, alcoholic beverages caused rectal bleeding. My doctor, using my x-ray as a chart, patiently explained why alcohol could not cause rectal bleeding! I will waste no more time on the past.

> "I switched to whole wheat bread and brown rice and started drinking freshly-squeezed orange juice every day. After some time, I realized that I no longer had diarrhea and was apparently absent of the symptoms of my disease. My doctor had warned me that, as an ulcerative colitis patient, my chances of contracting cancer of the colon were 20 percent higher than the average person.

"He recommended yearly x-rays to keep a close watch of the disease. When my daughter was 2½ years old, I decided it was time to check it. After the x-rays had been developed ... I wish I had a tape recorder to record his amazement. The diseased area was completely healed. No activity! He is a brilliant doctor who is connected with a major hospital (teaching) in New York City. How come I know something that he does not? He is supposed to be the expert!"

Tomato For Diarrhea!

Fresh dried tomato pulp in a pectin base is a well-known remedy for diarrhea. This combination is used in a drug called *Tomectin*.

> The successful use of tomato pomace in more than 100 cases of diarrhea is described by Lester M. Morrison, M.D., of the Philadelphia General Hospital, in the *American Journal of Digestive Diseases* (12:196, 1946). Dr. Morrison says that diarrhea from simple causes or non-organic causes was usually stopped within four hours by the tomato treatment!

In cases of food poisoning, allergy, malnutrition, and spastic colitis, diarrhea was relieved within 12 hours of the first dose. In all cases, milk with a tablespoon of the tomato pomace was given every two hours.

Like most other herbs and vegetables, tomato is best eaten fresh. Canned or cooked, it loses most of its nutrient value. Fresh tomato or tomato juice is alkaline. When combined with starch or sugar in the same meal, it becomes acid and will cause heartburn (as when taken with crackers on an empty stomach).

Diarrhea Ceased Almost Immediately!

Mrs. K.V. reports: "I had diarrhea for a long time, and was so weak I could hardly move. I felt exhausted and my weight dropped alarmingly. Every time I stopped taking the doctor's prescription, the diarrhea came back, worse than ever. Then I was told to try garlic, by taking a teaspoonful of the diced pieces with milk or honey, two or three times a day. The amazing thing is, my diarrhea ceased almost immediately!"

Garlic Therapy In Diseases Of The Digestive Tract!

E.E. Marcovici, M.D., in an article entitled, "Garlic Therapy in Diseases of the Digestive Tract Based on 25 Years' Experience" (*Practical Therapeutics*, January 15, 1941), reports that he first became interested in garlic in 1915 when, as an army physician, he had the opportunity of studying and treating innumerable cases of gastrointestinal infections, including dysentery and cholera.

Dr. Marcovici found that garlic brought speedy relief from the extreme diarrhea of dysentery. Some patients objected to the strong and pungent taste of the plant, so garlic tablets were used with equally good results. Results were so remarkable that garlic was later introduced as a routine treatment and cleansing measure in hundreds of cases of digestive disorders.

In chronic hypertension of the aged, Dr. Marcovici believes that garlic brings good results because of its cleansing effect on intestinal germs that cause putrefaction. It thereby prevents these poisons from being absorbed by the bloodstream.

"These patients are known to suffer frequently from chronic constipation, cecal stasis (intestinal blockage) or chronic appendicitis," he explains. "As a result of these disorders, foodstuffs incompletely predigested in the stomach on account of subacidity or hyperacidity, reach the cecal region where they undergo pathological putrefaction. As a consequence, toxins are absorbed and carried into the blood stream. This toxemia is responsible for the varying symptoms from which these patients suffer: headaches (migraine), dizziness, fatigue, capillary spasms, etc." Garlic kills germs of putrefaction to cleanse and purify the system.

Garlic For Diarrhea!

Dr. E. Roos, writing in *Munchener Medizinische Wochenschrift,* a German medical magazine, dated September 25, 1925 tells how he used a garlic preparation with success in treating many intestinal ailments, mostly involving diarrhea. He states that garlic is effective three ways: it soothes, cleanses and reduces inflammation. Garlic, he says, has an almost narcotic effect. Like a narcotic, it seems to make stomach aches, diarrhea, and other intestinal ailments disappear within a very short time. Unlike narcotics, garlic rarely causes constipation.

"It makes little difference," says Dr. Roos, "what kind of diarrhea you are dealing with or where it principally has its origin. A favorable result has been obtained in the great majority of cases treated, even in stubborn, chronic cases with recurrence."

Although results cannot be guaranteed, he says, in cases of serious organic disorder such as cancer or tuberculosis, he goes on to give several examples of seemingly hopeless cases treated with success. (The names in these cases have been changed.)

Reported Cases:
- A professor, Milton F., had suffered from gas, dyspepsia, and colitis for 17 years. Occasionally, the diarrhea alternated with spells of constipation. He was given two grams of the garlic preparation two to three times daily. In two and a half months the patient considered himself cured.
- Mrs. Odetta S., 59, suffered from diarrhea for almost nine months. Before that she had always been constipated—with a very sensitive and delicate digestive system. At the end of a month, with garlic treatment, she gained weight, appeared healthy, and her stools were completely normal. Evidence of large deposits of harmful bacteria in her intestines completely disappeared.
- Lucas R., 33, a churchman, suffered from chronic colitis, involving much pain and abdominal discomfort. He began by taking two grams of garlic twice a day for 14 days, then only daily. Within the first few days he felt better. Three weeks later, he had two normal bowel movements daily.
- Lena H., 24, suddenly experienced terrific body pain, nausea, chills and fever, along with persistent diarrhea. Her condition was diagnosed as acute enterocolitis. She took two grams of garlic three times a day, and by the fifth day her condition was perfectly normal.
- Clifford P., 49, a master baker, suffered from intense pressure pains in his upper abdomen. The pain had bothered him for more than a year, sometimes all day long—and yet he did not suffer from gas. He was given two tablets of garlic three times a day—and in a matter of days he experienced great improvement. In about a month, he declared himself in perfect health.
- Irwin W., a scholar, troubled with abdominal pains, stomach trouble, hyperacidity and diarrhea, was scheduled for an appendectomy. As luck would have it, the surgeon was not available. In the meantime, he was

given the garlic preparation, two grams twice daily. After a few days, he claimed he felt perfectly well, and the operation was cancelled. (Dr. Roos gives this example just to show garlic's soothing influence, not recommending it as a substitute for needed surgery.)

"Often, after a very short time," notes Dr. Roos, "the difficulties improve, the patients feel relieved and look better. ... So far as our patients could later tell, the effect also seems to last." He recommends two tablets of garlic three times daily as the best possible daily dose of intestinal complaints; in severe cases, two tablets five times daily and in light cases, two tablets once or twice daily. Most important of all, he notes these tablets can be taken without any fear of disagreeable side effects.

How Best To Take Garlic For Diarrhea!

Ms. H.L., of Bethesda, Maryland, gives these helpful hints on how to take garlic for diarrhea:

> "I have been subject at times to a persistent diarrhea," she states. "The various medications given me by my doctor did nothing for it, and made me feel sicker. I finally tried taking raw garlic after each meal and the diarrhea ceased immediately.

"Evidently," she continues, "it was caused by too many unfriendly bacteria which the garlic killed. I don't like chewing garlic so I chopped it fine and swallowed it with fruit juice."

As Gentle As A Kitten—Pleasing To The Taste When Used Correctly!

How often have you heard this complaint? "I ate some grated garlic and my stomach became so upset that I thought I would die." This is almost always due to improper use of garlic. Used correctly garlic is delicious and has no odor.

The way to really tame garlic is to cook it! This gives it a smooth, buttery texture, and a delicious nut-flavored taste. And the finished dish has no garlic odor at all! This is true even in certain exotic cooked dishes calling for as many as 60 cloves! The reason is that the essence (or odor) of garlic is a volatile oil that rapidly escapes in heat.

Cooked garlic, says one expert, is safe and flavorful—as are small amounts fresh, diced in salads or meat—and he recommends these for people in poor health, or with allergies or stomach ailments.[1] It is in large, raw doses that some people find garlic most upsetting. For such people it should always be diluted in some way, as in soup or with milk and crackers.

An Effective Remedy For Constipation!

Hippocrates recommended garlic as a highly effective laxative. A leading scientist and expert on garlic therapy states that people who suffer from constipation can find relief by regularly eating moderate amounts of garlic mixed with onions and milk or yogurt. The allicin in garlic, he says, stimulates peristaltic motion of the intestinal walls and in this way produces bowel movement. Kristine Nolfi, M.D., a Danish naturopathic physician also states that "Garlic has a strengthening and laxative effect."

Recovery Occurs In Minutes!

Garlic is unusually rich in potassium—529 mg. in 100 grams. Potassium is essential to the contraction of every muscle in the body. Without it, contractions of the intestinal muscles slow down markedly—these muscles may even become partially or completely paralyzed. This results in constipation!

---

[1] Tadashi Watanabe, D.Sc. *Garlic Therapy*, Japan Publications, Tokyo, 1974.

"Even though muscles become weak, lax, soft, or partially paralyzed, recovery occurs within minutes after potassium is taken," says one expert. Garlic, therefore, as a rich source of potassium may well explain its claimed effectiveness in cases of constipation.

Other sources of potassium include fruits and vegetables. Cooking fruits and vegetables brings about great losses in potassium—as does salting them. A low salt, high protein diet rich in potassium can usually prevent a deficiency.

9

Miracle Medicine Foods
For Eyes, Ears, Nose And Throat

The old motherly notion that eating carrots will give you blue eyes may not be accurate, but eye doctors have discovered that what you eat may affect how you see. For 20 years, eye specialists at Wills Eye Hospital in Philadelphia and Harvard's Retina Center in Cambridge, Massachusetts, and other scientists specializing in the correction and cure of defective vision have been aware of the connection between diet and failing eyesight.

> **"There's no sense damaging your eyes with your mouth," says Dr. Arthur Keeney, a Kentuckian who heads the staff at Wills. Keeney explained that the eye—particularly the sensitive area in the middle of the retina known as the macula—is very sensitive to changes stemming from a high-fat diet.**

In fact, he says, placing a patient on a low-fat diet is one means eye doctors have of controlling a mysterious but common visual defect known as macular degeneration, which deprives the individual of the ability to see straight ahead. In most cases irreversible, it is due to a blockage or leak in the tiny blood vessels which interlace the macula (a round light-sensitive spot at the center of the retina). The victim finds himself going blind in the central area of sight. Diet may help. In many eye ailments, miracle medicine foods seem to have helped!

Reported Cases:

- In one reported case, a 60-year-old man suffered from glaucoma for several years. During the last year, his eyesight was so bad he could only see shadows. On a friend's advice, he began eating three carrots a day boiled in about a quart of water. He drank all the water and used no seasoning. In nine days, he began to regain some eyesight. After using the carrots for two months, he can see shapes and colors, and identified a friend's Volkswagen parked across the street from his house!
- Mr. D.R. reports: "My eyesight was so weak, I could not read a printed page. Even large letters were blurry. My doctor said it was old age and poor circulation. Soon I was wearing thick lenses and using a magnifying glass. When I heard how raw liquid lecithin cleans out the bloodstream, I started taking 3 tablespoons a day. In two weeks, my vision cleared up. My doctor only shrugged and smiled. Why didn't he tell me this?"
- Ms. E.M. writes: "I was dangerously close to glaucoma with an eye pressure on the Tonameter of 17 and 21. A reading of 25 is glaucoma. My eye doctor advised me to cut my coffee which I failed to do. Around this time I started taking vitamins A, C and E and also bone meal. I was almost afraid to go back and have my eyes tested but I had to get my glasses changed. The doctor was shocked that my eye pressure had dropped to a reading of 15 and 14. I had lowered it a total of nine points and he said this is excellent. It was then that I told him I take lots of vitamins. He said vitamin C is the one vitamin that lowers eye pressure. My distance vision has improved so much."

A Word On Glaucoma!

It is extremely important not to attempt to treat glaucoma yourself by dietary measures alone without your doctor's approval, for this disease has several forms.[1] If simple dietary measures, such as a reduction in fluid intake, and eyedrops to relieve pressure inside the eye, do not work, a simple operation is performed to relieve the pressure and save the sight. Some researchers believe there is a connection between glaucoma and lack of vitamins A, B, and C. Many doctors also believe coffee should be avoided.

How Cataracts Melted Away!

Cataract is a loss of transparency of the crystalline lens of the eye. It, too, has several forms—one in which the lens is hardened and of a deep brown color, another in which it is green (glaucoma), other forms in which it is gray or milky, or affecting only part of the eye, perhaps with scarring or skin disease—in all, several dozen forms, which only a doctor can diagnose. In the most common form, vision becomes blurry, like a frosted glass window, and there is profuse tearing and irritation.

> Almost 100 percent cures have been reported for cataracts, using vitamin B-2 therapy. Marked healing occurred in 24 to 48 hours. Vision cleared and burning, itching, redness and tearing were gone, using 15 milligrams of B-2 daily, and nothing else. Subjects were completely cured with this Miracle Medicine Food.

These amazing results were reported by Dr. Sydenstricker of the University of Georgia, testing 24 patients, 18 of whom had a noticeable white coating on their eyes (beginning sign of cataract). All the others had advanced cataracts. To see if it was the vitamin B-2—and nothing else—that cured them, a few volunteers were asked to stop taking it. Cataracts began forming. These quickly disappeared when this miracle medicine food, vitamin B-2, was supplied in tablet form. Common foods containing vitamin B-2 include calf liver,

---

[1] Glaucoma patients who self-treat run the risk of blindness, for this disease has several forms, the most dangerous being glaucoma fulminans, which can literally wipe out vision overnight.

broccoli, raw collards, turnip tops, beets, wheat germ, peanuts, brewer's yeast, chicken, salmon, nuts and beans.

> **Vitamin C is often mentioned in connection with cataracts—sufferers often lack it. In experiments with laboratory animals upon whom cataracts had been induced, the growth of cataracts was inhibited by increasing vitamin C intake.**

In *Eye, Ear, Nose and Throat Monthly* (volume 31), a doctor says that his method for preventing or correcting cataracts is to give his patients a special diet which includes the tops of vegetables—which I call garlic foods (foods that go well with garlic). They also get a pint of milk and two eggs daily, with vitamin C and A and chlorophyll tablets. Calcium is also often mentioned in connection with cataracts. Apparently, a lack of calcium allows cataracts to form. Foods rich in calcium include common beans, beet greens, watercress, dandelion greens, mustard greens, parsley, and turnip greens. (All contain roughly 200 mg. per serving.)

Reported Cases:
- Mrs. W.M. reports: "I became interested in natural supplement 4½ years ago when my 90-year-old grandmother learned she was going blind from cataracts (dimming vision, red, weepy eyes and a noticeable film). She began taking vitamins A, B-2, C, D, and E, dessicated liver, sunflower seed meal, organex and protein. At 94, the cataracts are gone and her mental and physical health have improved tremendously. (Take care of your body and your eyes will take care of themselves?)"
- Mr. M.A. reports: "Three years ago my E.E.N.T. specialist told me he would have to remove cataracts from both eyes. I began taking vitamins A and B complex, together with yeast and liver, about three grams of C each day, kelp, dolomite, bone meal, and other calcium tablets, lecithin, and pantothenic acid.... The cataracts are gradually disappearing and I can see much better."

- Mrs. W.M. writes: "My grandmother was told she was developing cataracts and would, eventually, have to have an operation to save her sight.... After considerable persuasion, she agreed to try the supplements which I suggested. We started her on vitamins A, C, B, and bone meal. This was two years ago and grandma's general health has improved considerably, and her eyesight has improved to the point where she sits and plays cards with us and has no more 'weeping' which had caused her so much discomfort."
- One man writes: "My eyes were very painful ... a film gathering over them." He remembered reading about the medicinal value of olive oil. This he applied to his eyes and eyelids, also beneath the eyes and under the eyelids. He claimed that after two or three applications, his sight was entirely restored!
- Another man says: "I had a horse going blind with a white film over his eyes, which seemed to hurt. His eyes was shut and watered. I dipped white honey into his eyes with a feather for several nights. In a day or so the film was gone and the eye looked bright and good."

Corneal Ulcers Relieved!

The *British Medical Journal*, November 18, 1950, says that in 51 cases of small corneal ulcers of the eye, half the patients were given vitamin C (1500 mg.) and half received a placebo, of no medicinal value. In those who received the vitamin C, the deep ulcers healed rapidly!

A Dutch scientific journal on botanical medicine[2] says: "*Hydrastis* (golden seal) tincture or fluid extract applied externally to the cornea in a dilution of two drops in an eye bath will heal a corneal ulcer if used three times daily."

Finally, severe ulcers of the cornea of the eye have been treated with good results by injections of vitamin C—and

---
[2] *Acta Phytotherapeutica*, XII: 9.

large amounts have been suggested when cataract is present, according to the *American Journal of Ophthalmology*, June 1951.

Food For Near and Distant Vision!

Vitamin A is essential to good vision. A mild deficiency makes it difficult to see at night. A more severe form results in headaches from bright light. Burning, itching and a gritty sensation under the eyelids may develop. In advanced stages, pus and ulcers may form—and dark spots may appear before the eyes (scotomata).

Myopia or nearsightedness may be due to a lack of calcium and vitamin A in the diet, according to the *American Journal of Ophthalmology*, May 1950. The AMA recommends about 5,000 units of vitamin A daily —10-15 times as much in cases of deficiency. Common foods rich in vitamin A include cooked chard, dandelion leaves and beet greens. A four-ounce serving of these contains 15,000 to 20,000 units of vitamin A. These foods are also rich in calcium. Other good sources include watercress, kale, mustard greens, turnip greens and parsley.

Sunflower seeds have been found to relieve farsightedness, eye strain, ache and pain, and extreme light sensitivity, such as the bright reflection from snow or the glare from automobile headlights and TV screens. Sunflower seeds contain 50 units of vitamin A per 100 grams, and are also rich in B complex vitamins, iron and calcium.

Reported Cases:
- Mr. H.B. Reports: "Sunflower seeds have done a lot of good for me. I needed reading glasses since I was 45 years old, am 65 now, have eaten the seeds for about two years or more and can read a lot now without glasses."
- Mrs. F.N. writes: "I brought my eyesight back with sunflower seeds, three teaspoonfuls of the kernels a

day. Everything was a blur, but now I can read without glasses. Even my hair is getting life and luster back into it."

- Mrs. S.G. reports: "Having had severe eye trouble for many years I decided to try (sunflower) seeds. I ate a good-sized handful each day and in about two weeks I noticed a definite and almost unbelievable change. The strain, ache, and pain almost completely disappeared and I could work the entire day without being conscious of any trouble. An eye specialist (one of the best), after an examination, stated that my eyes had improved, and he prescribed weaker lenses."

- Mr. J.S. states: "The very first time I ate sunflower seeds I felt results! I knew then and there that sunflower seeds were good for me and something my eyes needed. And the more I have eaten, the better they get. The results are immediate and at the same time lasting."

- Mrs. O.B. writes: "I am 66 years old and have always worn glasses. Have unusually far vision, so objects near were hard to distinguish.... I have never taken vitamins in any amount. I use about half a cup of sunflower seeds a day. I eat while ironing, walking, while on the bus or while reading or listening to the radio. I can at times thread a needle and sew without the aid of glasses. Often go all day without glasses, which I have not been able to do for many years.... I feel the seeds are really helping me to restore my eyesight."

The Vitamin In Garlic That Restored Sight!

Finally, there is the thiamin-boosting ingredient which garlic contains, increasing the body's absorption of B-1 (thiamin) tenfold!

This vitamin is vital to eye and nerve health. Dimness of vision, impairment of the field of vision, blackouts, inability to focus or see up close ("amblyopia")—caused

by too much alcohol and tobacco—have been corrected with B-1, as follows.

F.D. Carroll, in the *American Journal of Ophthalmology* (June 1945), tells of a case in which about half of the patient's calories came from alcohol, and his consumption of B vitamins was considered inadequate. Without decreasing tobacco or alcohol consumption, or improving the diet, normal vision was restored by administering 40 mg. of thiamin per day by mouth, and 20 by vein. Improvement was maintained as long as the patient took 10 mg. tablets of thiamin a day. Without them, vision became impaired.

Spots Before The Eyes Can Clear Up!

Reportedly, spots before the eyes can also be relieved with B vitamins. Such spots are nothing more than "floaters" —small particles moving inside the eyes. Ordinarily, you never see them. But when eyes become fatigued, as in the case of lack of B vitamins, the optic nerves become so jumpy that even those shadows are noticed.

> Robert B. thought that he was going blind, when he began to see large spots before his eyes. He couldn't read or watch television or concentrate on anything—even looking out the window on a bright, sunny day was spoiled for him because of annoying spots that seemed to travel as his eyes moved—or settled—directly in his line of vision.

He described these spots to his doctor. They had strange shapes and looked like germs in a microscope. Most were transparent, but some were splotchy and a little darker. His doctor told him not to worry—that these were just pigments or colored particles floating inside the eyeball. He told Robert that if he should ever see a dark black spot, that might be serious and he should get it checked—but that these floaters would go away, there was nothing to do but wait it out.

Then Robert read that B vitamins were healing to the nerves, the optic nerves in particular, and that garlic increased their absorption tenfold. Reasoning that a good garlic food program might erase these spots, he began to eat garlic with foods rich in B vitamins. Two days later, he suddenly noticed the spots were gone! He continues to follow the garlic food program. His vision is perfect, and the problem never returned!

Eye "Floaters" Vanish!

Mr. R.N. reports: "For about four years I had considerable trouble with spots (floaters) behind my eyes. After seeing an optometrist I was told they would probably always bother me, so I more or less resigned myself to this annoying problem. Then about four months ago I decided to treat myself for a sinus headache with vitamin C. I took two grams every hour for about 16 hours. The headache disappeared overnight and I realized at the same time that the spots in my eyes had disappeared as well. I haven't had a sign of them since."

Glaucoma Symptoms Vanished!

Mrs. B.E. reports: "I am 36 years old, too young to have glaucoma, most doctors think. In fact, few even test for it. I was lucky; mine did. A year ago, the pressure was up to 36 in one eye, and 32 in the other eye. I tried drops and found they not only did not lower the pressure, but that they irritated my eyes.

"The doctor said we could try a stronger drop, but I refused. Three months ago I decided to try vitamins. I have used 2,000 to 3,000 mg. of vitamin C with rose hips plus 150 mg. of rutin twice a day for three months. Last week my pressures were taken again and they were normal (20). My eye doctor wouldn't believe it. I told him about my vitamins and he is so interested he is going to tell his other glaucoma patients." Others report the same results.

Eye Miraculously Healed By Common Herb

The common herb, comfrey, seems to possess extraordinary healing powers when used as a poultice or tea drink. Doctors have used its medicinal extract, *allantoin,* in cases of stubborn ulcers, burns, and open wounds, with spectacular results!

An eye doctor was astonished when a patient, suffering a deep burn of the eyeball—due to red hot molten copper which had splashed on him—was miraculously healed by a liquid derived from the common herb comfrey. The swelling of the cornea disappeared, with firm healing of deeper layers and the formation of new tissue, described as rapid and dramatic!

Many Near-Blind Cases Helped!

Reportedly, many cases of near blindness have been helped by nerve massage. For eye weakness, massage the pads at the base of the second and third fingers on both hands, left hand for left eye, right hand for right eye. Pressure on the ends of these fingers can relieve eye strain in a few minutes. To stop watering eyes, massage the webs between these fingers. An elderly woman with cataracts used this miracle medicine food for the eyes. In a short time, her near-blindness was relieved to the point where she was able to read, and no longer had to be led around!

Hearing Can be Improved Up to 90%

You can also use this method to help bring back hearing, says one expert. Press the tip of the third, or ring finger, for about 5 minutes, several times a day (left hand for left ear, right hand for right ear). Pressure on the joints of this finger and the little finger may also help. There are doctors who claim up to 90 percent improvement, in almost all cases of deafness due to thickening of the ear membrane, ear noises, and ringing in the ears. Everyone obtains some benefit, says one expert. One man who was deaf for 25 years, and could hardly hear loud talking, used this miracle medicine food—in five minutes he could hear a whisper across a room! Another man, almost totally deaf, used it and in ten minutes he could hear the ticking of his car's directional signals, children's voices, the TV—without a hearing aid, for the first time!

Miracle Medicine Foods For The Ears!

Miracle medicine foods may well ease your hearing problems. *Medical World News* tells the story of Dr. J.T. Spencer, Jr. of Charleston, W. Va., who suffered from progressive hearing loss and occasional dizziness. But after going on a low cholesterol and low carbohydrate diet (for an allergy problem), he suddenly found that much of his hearing returned. He tested the same approach on some of his patients (he's an ear specialist) and says many have improved hearing.

Sudden deafness requires immediate medical attention, due to its many possible causes—such as Ménière's Disease, certain types of infection, a blood clot, poor circulation, or other causes. In the *Journal of the American Medical Association*, November 30, 1957, Dr. O. Erick Hallberg writes that hardening of the arteries can lead to an insufficient supply of blood to the inner ear, thereby causing sudden deafness.

Deafness from an insufficient blood supply is fairly constant, with ringing in the ears and dizziness, he says, while other types of deafness may come and go. It is not likely to affect both ears at once. In discussing the general treatment of deafness due to hardening of the arteries, Dr. Hallberg says: "The continuing use of nicotinic acid (a B vitamin) in high dosage seems to be most beneficial both for its vasodilating (artery widening) effect and also for its apparent tendency to reduce the blood cholesterol level. Patients should also be put on a low fat diet and should stay on it the rest of their lives." Foods that contain the B vitamins include liver, wheat germ, and brewer's yeast. Dr. Hallberg also mentions the addition of unsaturated vegetable oils to the diet as a means of lowering the cholesterol level of the blood. Two of the best are olive oil and soybean oil (which contains the important fat dissolver, lecithin).

Reported Cases:
- **A doctor, age 40, suddenly noticed a blurred sensation in his left ear. He had no head cold or dizziness, but he felt there was something in his ear. An examination showed no blockage of any kind; however, an audiogram showed a sharp hearing loss on that side. Blood tests revealed a high fat level. He was put on a low fat diet (lean meats, fresh fruits and vegetables—no butter, eggs, cream, gravy, starches, or processed cheeses). In two weeks, his hearing returned to normal!**
- **Mr. J.D. complained of deafness and a ringing noise in his ear for many years. When he began to use lots of soybean lecithin every day, suddenly the ringing stopped and his hearing cleared! He is so happy that he plans to keep using this miracle medicine food that improves circulation and cleans out fat-encrusted veins and arteries, causing sudden hearing improvement in many cases!**

Other Ear Problems Relieved With Miracle Medicine Foods!

Ms. L.C. reports: "For one year I have used garlic oil for earaches. I have seen it work wonders within ten to 15 minutes of puncturing a garlic oil capsule, pouring it into the ear and stopping it with a little cotton. I have told friends and relatives about how the pain stops soon after, and they all swear by it!

"My sister had an inner ear infection and cried all through the night with pain. She called me at 4:00 a.m. in tears. Her husband came and got some oil, and the pain was relieved in 15 minutes. Also, I found quite by accident that burns are helped by garlic oil rubbed into the burn. The pain goes away almost immediately upon application and rubbing it into the burn.

"My nephew burned his hand quite badly on top of the electric stove. When garlic oil was applied, he was very much relieved, and slept through the night without crying."

Ringing Ears Relieved!

Mr. S.A. reports: "I have discovered a very simple and cheap remedy for bad hearing and ringing in the ears.... My ears would ring so much and my hearing was very cloudy. Three years ago I read, 'It is said that a drop of onion juice in the ear is good for bad hearing.' I tried it with wonderful results. Start about three times a week and as your condition improves you may cut down. I now use it about every week or ten days and maintain good results."

The Herb With The Miracle Healing Power!

A medical doctor reports the case of a man with a large tumor in his nose and mouth, which was removed surgically. A month later, the growth had again returned. It bulged through the incision and almost closed the right eye. It was blue, firm and did not break. His case was hopeless, and he was sent home to die.

A few weeks later, the patient walked into the doctor's office looking in better health than he had ever been. The tumor had completely disappeared from the face and there was no trace of it in the mouth. He had no pain and was apparently well.

He told the doctor he had treated it by applying poultices of comfrey and the swelling had gradually disappeared. The doctor stated that he did not believe that such a thing was possible. (As in all cases involving the eye, ear, nose and throat, the reader is cautioned to seek immediate medical care. Self-treatment is not recommended, unless your doctor approves.)

Horrible Throat Pain Relieved!

One of these miracle medicine foods is so powerful that —while not a cure—it has been used to relieve the horrible pains of throat cancer. It is a well-known fact that sufferers have said that only violet leaf tea, used as a drink, mouthwash or gargle, relieved their agony. Use of this common tea is not permitted without a doctor's approval. It is no substitute for qualified medical care.

Sore Tongue Remedy!

Mrs. A.T. reports: "My tongue frequently felt sore, and it was very annoying. Two physicians disregarded my complaint since there was no visible sign of irritation. But when I asked my dentist about it, he asked whether I was on a special diet. I was—for an ulcer, which naturally meant no fresh fruit. He suggested that scurvy was beginning and told me to take big doses of vitamin C. The awful misery was gone in a couple of days!"

Rx For A Burning Tongue!

The *Journal of the American Medical Association* (January 1, 1976) reports that a burning tongue, usually involving both sides, and often accompanied by a dry or sore throat, is a common complaint in menopausal or older women. Lack of hydrochloric acid in the stomach is a frequent cause, in which case doctors give an acid stimulant. In patients with normal stomach acid, a liver supplement is prescribed, along with vitamin B-12 and riboflavin. Reportedly, most patients are relieved by these treatments.

Miracle Medicine Food For The Nose and Throat!

Garlic has long been known as a miracle antiseptic in cases involving eye, ear, nose and throat infection. As Kristine Nolfi, M.D., states:[3]

> "If one puts a piece of garlic in his mouth, at the onset of a cold, on both sides between cheek and teeth, the cold will disappear within a few hours or, at most, within a day!

Garlic also has a curative effect on chronic diseases in the upper respiratory organs, the doctor says, absorbing the poisons—and this is true for "chronic inflammation of the tonsils, salivary glands and neighboring lymph glands, empyema of the maxillary sinus, severe pharyngitis and laryngitis" and other conditions. For example:

- This miracle healing plant, says the doctor, "makes loose teeth take root again, removes tartar!"
- It has a curative effect on eye catarrh and inflammation of the lacrymal (tear) duct!
- Got an earache? Just wrap the plant in some gauze, says the doctor, and place it in the outer ear canal!
- Got a headache? Garlic is nature's aspirin, dilating the veins and arteries to relieve congestion. Just squeeze some garlic juice into a teaspoon of honey (it's an old American Indian remedy)!
- Sneezing, stuffy nose or allergy got you down? Try a little diced garlic downed with water. Garlic reportedly works miracles in such cases!

Treating Colds With Garlic!

Dr. J. Klosa experimented with garlic and reported his findings in an issue of the German magazine *Medical Month-*

---

[3]*My Experiences With Living Food*, by Kristine Nolfi, M.D. Humlegaarden, Humleback, Denmark, n.d.

ly, March 1950. Dr. Klosa experimented with a specially prepared solution of garlic oil and water (two grams of garlic oil to one kilogram of water).

> In 71 cases, clogged and running noses completely cleared up in 13 to 20 minutes! Burning and tickling in the throat could be stopped immediately by administering 30 drops of the oil of garlic solution—if symptoms were caught in the first stage. Otherwise, they abated to the point of disappearance in 24 hours!

Dr. Klosa reports the results with grippe, sore throat, and rhinitis (clogged and running nose) patients. The fever and catarrhal symptoms of 13 cases of grippe were cut short in every case. Cough symptoms were suppressed. Not one of the patients suffered from the usual post-grippe complaints such as swelling of the lymph glands, jaundice, pains in muscles or joints, or chronic inflammation of the lungs. All patients show a definite lessening of the required period of convalescence! The usual dosage was 10 to 25 drops taken partly by mouth and partly by being administered directly into the nostrils every four hours.

Garlic For Sore Throat!

Garlic works faster than vitamin C in curing colds. If one keeps a clove of garlic in the mouth, the cold will disappear within a few hours, or at most half a day, in my experience. It will not burn at all unless you chew it. Just score it with your teeth, every so often, to release a little juice. (If garlic is too strong, try one of its milder cousins like rocambole or sand leek.)

> In this manner, a sore throat can be stopped in *minutes* (it even works for dreaded sore throat symptoms of diphtheria)! I have found it to work every time—and to be much more reliable than vitamin C, which may or may not work, and often only forestalls the inevitable. Garlic gives permanent, not just temporary relief.

It is a lot simpler than vitamin C, which must be taken in large doses, 500 mg. every two hours (according to F. Klenner, M.D.) or up to 1,000 mg. *an hour* (according to Dr. Linus Pauling), and takes up to 48 hours to work.

Garlic For Sinus!

Mrs. L.E. reports: "I wish to let you know what wonderful results I had with garlic, to clear up an attack of sinus. Normally, when my little daughter begins to have a fever (about twice a year), headaches and dizziness, I rush her off to the doctor—which usually costs me about $7 plus sinus medication of some sort. This last time she began to get sick, I had just read about how good garlic is for infections and colds, so I decided to try it. I bought garlic (with chlorophyll) and gave her two tablets about every four hours. After about six tablets, she woke up the next morning with a clear head and felt fine. All signs of sinus congestion were gone."

Receding Gums and Loose Teeth Firm Up Again!

Mr. S.C. reports: "Ever since I was 13 (I am now past 61), I have been troubled with a gum problem—the result of tartar accumulation under the gum line. This condition in turn would cause 'pockets' where the gum would recede from the tooth, probably resulting in a domino effect such as gum bleeding, puffiness and in some instances, loosened teeth.

"The only remedy open to such individuals as myself was to utilize the services of a very competent dentist who would regularly 'scale' my teeth at and below the gum line to remove tartar accumulation. On one occasion, surgery was employed to cut away tissue pockets in order to promote gum healing. This routine was standard procedure for me on approximately a twice a year basis.

"About six months ago I quite casually began taking 250 mg. of vitamin C daily, because I'd heard it was good for colds. On my last visit to the dentist a week ago, he remarked how my gums had become firm and that his instruments could hardly go below the gum line. He said I must really be doing a good job with my toothbrush. I don't think so. I think it was the vitamin C, which was the only big change in my diet."[4]

Excruciating Tooth and Gum Pain Relieved Instantly!

Miss G.C. reports: "About three weeks ago my dentist pulled my top wisdom tooth. . . . He gave me some codeine pills and sent me home.

"A few days later that side of my mouth hurt so badly I was almost hysterical; my mother mixed me some epsom salt and hot water, had me gargle on the left side of my mouth with it quite a few times and keep spitting it out. It worked like magic for me!

"Every time the pain started coming back, I used more epsom salt and hot water. After about a day, all pain was *completely gone*. Anybody with wisdom tooth pains, *try it! It works!*"

Bleeding Gums Healed!

Miss L. W. reports: "My gums have been bleeding horribly for at least seven years. I have been through several dentists, lots of dental work, and loads of money, but nothing has helped. For other reasons, I started taking 20 mg. of zinc and 500 mg. of vitamin C daily about 1½ months ago. Last night I noticed I was vigorously brushing my teeth (I mean really scrubbing them!). I was amazed and had to sit down and think about really brushing my teeth for the first time that I can remember in ages! It had to be a result of zinc or vitamin C, but what? I remember reading somewhere how a man with bleeding gums accidentally cured them

---

[4]Garlic may be good for gum infection. One doctor stated: "Garlic, for some unknown reason, seems to have an affinity for pus pockets. This is probably due to its high organic sulfur content which acts as an antiseptic cleansing mineral."

with vitamin C. Amazing! I just can't believe it. After years of hassling—just like that—the condition is completely gone!"

Miracle Medicine Foods Save Teeth!

Mrs. L.R. reports: "For quite some time I have suffered from extreme gum problems. A periodontist wanted to pull all but a few of my teeth as a solution. Being not too old (30) I felt there had to be another solution.

"I found a periodontist who felt he could save my teeth and that my problem was definitely systemic. The first thing he did was to send off a sample of my hair along with a questionnaire and blood sample to a lab. The results came back—I was extremely low in almost every important mineral and some trace elements—all working (or not working) to cause deterioration of bones, infections of gums, etc.

"After taking supplements for several months now, I still have my teeth, my general health has improved, and best of all my gum problem seems to have improved. The dentist also recommends a diet of natural foods and lots of vitamin C—all together it certainly seems to work!"

10

Miracle Medicine Foods For Hay Fever And Allergies!

In Vermont, honey is used for treating hay fever. If the pollen that causes it can be discovered, the sufferer is fed honey made from that pollen. Also, hay fever victims are advised to chew on honeycombs for several months before and during the hay fever season, and to take honey mixed with apple cider vinegar three or four times a day. Reportedly, chewing honeycombs keeps the nasal passages open and acts as a sedative.

Reported Cases:
- For 25 years, one man reports he suffered from hay fever every June. Attacks started in the first week of June and ended in the first week of July. Upon hearing that honeycomb was recommended for hay fever, he purchased some and chewed on a teaspoonful during a severe attack. The hay fever vanished in seconds, and each time it recurred, the same simple remedy banished it!
- Mrs. F.O. reports: "My husband used to have bad hay fever. (Then a friend suggested honey), two tablespoons a day, starting one month before hay fever time, and on through. It really worked. He took shots and was in air conditioning. This is his second year without shots. Our daughter got it too. She would not try it at first. She did not like honey at all but takes it now. No

shots now. It is wonderful. It makes a difference in the honey, too. We use the fall honey."

Comfrey—The Green Miracle For Hay Fever!

Mrs. B.C. reports: "Several years ago, my grandfather, a lifelong hayfever sufferer, heard that comfrey was good for the treatment of allergies. He got hold of some roots and planted them in his garden.

"**From the time the plants are large enough to spare a few leaves, he begins eating two six-inch leaves a day—maybe three or four. This has completely controlled his hay fever. His sons, daughters, and myself have all tried the same remedy with the same results—a complete end to hay fever so long as comfrey is eaten throughout the season.**

"Before I was completely sold on it, I suffered for six weeks with drippy nose, itchy eyes, etc. It took about one week of eating comfrey each day to control it. In the middle of the summer, I got careless and quit eating it daily. After several days the symptoms returned. My return to comfrey helped again. Since the leaves are hairy we find that folding them up into small squares with the stem and top of the leaf to the inside makes them more palatable.

"Fresh leaves chewed very thoroughly are also supposed to be good for ulcers. Leaves brewed into a tea may be just as efficacious as the fresh leaves, but none of us have tried them that way for hay fever control or ulcers."

A Wonderful Remedy For Asthmatic Allergy Night Coughs!

"Quite by accident," Mrs. B.C. continues, "I discovered a marvelous remedy for those awful asthmatic, allergy coughs or children's hacky night coughs. My little girl awoke late one night coughing in a way that I was sure would keep us up with her all night long.

"I happened to have some comfrey tea on the stove that had been sitting there most of the day with the leaves still in it. About a quarter to half a cup with a teaspoon of honey to sweeten it had her back asleep in 15 minutes. That was the end of the coughing spell.

"Since then I recommended the treatment to two friends with asthmatic or allergic children. They can't believe how well it works! After sitting up so many nights with a coughing child who breathes only with difficulty, comfrey tea seems like a miracle.

"My uncle awoke with a severe cough one night and remembered what I'd said about comfrey. He went to his garden and got a few leaves, but chewed them slowly rather than brew a tea. The result was the same—he slept all night long. The power of a green plant is a miracle indeed!"

Another Man Swears By Comfrey!

Mr. S.M. writes: "Over the past seven years, I have invested a great deal of money in doctor bills and allergy treatments—all to no positive end. The most recent treatment made me extremely tired and induced drowsiness and sleep, making it impractical as a remedy during the work day.

"My mother introduced me to comfrey and comfrey tablets when brewing tea was not convenient. Since then I have at least two cups a day: one in the evening and one at mid-day. Relief has been permanent.

"There are no side effects and I prefer comfrey to commercial teas I purchased at my office. I strongly urge anyone suffering from hay fever or similar allergies to give comfrey a try. If your experience is close to mine, you are in for a pleasant and lasting surprise."

A Folklore Healer For Allergies!

The great French herbalist, Maurice Mességué, in *Of Men and Plants* gives a remedy for allergies in which garlic is a prime ingredient:

> Garlic (one crushed head)
> Single seed hawthorn (blossom—one handful)
> Greater celandine (flowers and stems, if possible, semi-fresh—one handful)
> Couch-grass (roots—one handful)
> Common broom (flowers—one handful)
> Sage (leaves—one handful)
> Linden (blossom—one handful)

This, he says, is to be used in foot- and hand-baths. (See instructions for basic preparations, page 37).[1]

The story is told of a European houseworker, Klara Y., who amazed her employers by rarely catching cold and resisting contagious diseases when others had serious bronchial disorders and winter ailments.

She said that it was a folklore remedy to chew and eat garlic daily to help build resistance to infections and act as a natural healer for respiratory or bronchial disorders. Other members of the household began taking this folklore healer and were able to heal their allergic symptoms.

As reported by Carlson Wade in *Magic Enzymes:* "The harmful effects of the virus organisms are inactivated and a healing power is experienced. For many Europeans, eating garlic is a natural way to help fight allergic disorders ranging from the common cold to bronchial spasms and attacks."[2]

---

[1] Reprinted with permission of Macmillan Publishing Co., Inc., from *Of Men and Plants* by Maurice Mességué. Copyright © 1972 by Weidenfeld & Nicolson Ltd. Copyright © 1973 by Macmillan Publishing Co., Inc.,
[2] Parker Publishing Company, Inc., 1973.

"Like A New Religious Experience!"

Mrs. A.S. reports: "The greatest thing ever to happen to me healthwise was... garlic! For years I have been plagued with stomach and respiratory problems. 'Allergies,' the doctors would say and drop the matter.

"I grew steadily worse until 11:00 p.m. became the most dreaded time of the day. When sleep would finally come I soon awakened almost drowning. I coughed, wheezed, and gasped for air. At 56, I threatened an early retirement.... I became an important customer of the drug companies who made antacids. These created other problems. Then I heard about garlic oil for allergies. I began taking 20 drops a day.

"The results are like a new religious experience. I was one who felt the difference in seven days. The comfort and ease I feel now is beyond description. All things being equal, I'll go the full route to retirement."

An Effective Remedy For Virus And Other Infections

Reportedly, an effective remedy for treating virus and other infections is six cloves of garlic. These can be chopped and added to green salad, or crushed and blended with butter and spread on bread (or toast). In addition, one should drink a glassful of hot water in which has been stirred four tablespoons of cider vinegar and two tablespoons of honey.

Near Fatal Attack Of Sneezing Relieved!

The story is told of a young man—we'll call him Harry I.—of Reno, Nevada, who had been sneezing for four days. Doctors tried everything, but nothing stopped the spasms.

Finally, a doctor who had read of the case in his local newspaper, suggested feeding the patient lots of garlic.

This was tried. Almost immediately, the patient stopped sneezing and fell into a restful sleep—his first since the attack!

"I believe the garlic cured him," said his physician. In another case, Carmella J., 21, of Oak Ridge, Tennessee, experienced an attack of almost continuous sneezing for six days. A diet of garlic halted the seizure. Her sneezing, which had been as rapid as 14 per minute, gradually subsided and finally stopped, when the garlic was eaten.

Hay Fever and Chronic Allergies Cured!

Phyllis S. suffered from hay fever and a whole raft of allergies that kept her sneezing, sniffling and miserable the year round. To look at her was to know she could hardly breathe. Her eyes were red and swollen and watery looking. She was constantly blowing her nose and sniffling through tons of tissues. The wheezing and continuous sneezing made it difficult for her to talk. She complained of a stuffed-up feeling that even prevented her from sleeping (she'd have to prop herself up with pillows—sitting bolt upright was the only way she could get any rest).

Phyllis was allergic to practically everything, including dogs, cats, grass, dust, pollen, ragweed, mould and spores. Her home was like a drugstore, filled with pills and sprays of every kind, which gave her only temporary relief with bad side effects like drowsiness, itching rashes and indigestion. She went to a whole series of doctors. One doctor told her to avoid chills and drafts and keep her neck warm (she was very susceptible to colds and suffered repeated infections that went from her nose to her throat to her lungs, with horrible attacks of bronchitis and a deep chest cough). Another doctor said she had nasal polyps, removed them in a painful operation, and they promptly grew back. Another doctor wanted to give her a series of allergy shots in a special three-year program, which she refused. "I'm so tired of a stuffed-up head, runny eyes, and a post-nasal drip," she said. "What I really need is a new body."

Then she discovered garlic, the miracle rejuvenation

plant, and the garlic food program with foods rich in vitamin C, and herbs including comfrey and elderberry teas that seemed to bring immediate relief. She tried the various garlic remedies, including the foot and hand baths. Within two weeks, she felt better than she had in years. Within a month, an allergy specialist gave her a clean bill of health. Her tests revealed no more allergies!

Amazing Relief For Hay Fever!

Onion, a mild form of garlic, is often used for dramatic relief of hay fever (caused by tree or rose pollen), in homeopathic medicine. In homeopathy, illness is treated by giving a person something—usually a plant or herb—that would produce his or her symptoms in a healthy person, in an attempt to "desensitize" the sufferer. In this way, immunity is gradually built up. This is the whole basis of vaccinations or innoculations for many diseases.

Hay fever is an allergy, and onion is an actual hay fever medicine. One medical doctor states: "I have found onion in high dilution to be my single most effective medication for spring and fall hay fever . . ."[3]

As onion is as close as your nearest grocery store, he states, you can readily prepare your own medication the homeopathic way! Just the way homeopathic physicians made their own medicine 100 years ago, before the development of our modern pharmacies!

A botanical medicine such as common onion (*Allium cepa*) is particularly easy to prepare at home, since its crushed leaves are soluble. A medicine is prepared by mixing one drop of the crushed pulp thoroughly in nine drops of a mixture of 87% ethyl alcohol and water. (Since you need a doctor's prescription to purchase pure ethyl alcohol, vodka would probably be the best substitute; you may also use brandy or

---

[3] James H. Stevenson, M.D., *A Homeopathic Doctor's Treasury of Health Secrets*, West Nyack, N.Y.; Parker Publishing Co., Inc., 1976.

whiskey. And you should do this in a nonbreakable glass bottle—you need six to twelve such bottles.) Add one drop of this to a second bottle, containing another nine drops of vodka mixed with water. Strike bottle #2 sharply 15 times against the palm of your hand, your shoe or thigh, or any other firm but soft object that won't shatter glass. Place one drop from bottle #2 into another clean bottle (#3), containing nine drops of the vodka and water mixture, and repeat the process. Continue in this manner from bottle to bottle until you have used either six or twelve bottles. *The last bottle in the series,* bottle #6 or 12, is the one you will use. (When the process has been repeated six times, you have a 6x dilution, and 12x means you've done it 12 times.) This may be kept in a light-resistant brown bottle with a neutral plastic, cork or glass top.

Reportedly, the usual dose is one drop from the final bottle in a glass of water. Take a sip and note its effect. If you are better, stop. If there has been no effect, take another sip in 3 hours, and repeat again in 3 hours if necessary. If you still see no change in your symptoms, try one sip each morning for a week. If no change occurs after a week, stop. And stop whenever you do notice an improvement—more than likely it will continue to improve. If you have a relapse, start all over again, immediately stopping as soon as you notice an improvement.[4]

Immediate Relief For Hangovers!

One doctor reports that most hangovers are caused by allergies! That is, the person is allergic—or extremely sensitive—to something in the drink, such as corn, rye or yeast. He found this to be true in nearly 20,000 cases. More amazing, he claims that a homeopathic dose of just *one drop* of

---

[4]Another method is simply to purchase this medicine from a homeopathic pharmacy all ready for instant use. Just ask for *Allium cepa* in the 6x or 12x dilution. Homeopathic medicines may be obtained from Ehrhart & Karl, Inc., 17 North Wabash Av., Chicago, Illinois 60602, and others. Some provide free catalogues. Pre-packaged homeopathic medicines often come in tablet form. Reportedly, they do not spoil—and a typical one dram bottle, costing $3 or $4, may last for years.

what you drank the night before—in a glass of water—can relieve your hangover almost immediately! Take 2 or 3 sips. If hangover symptoms, such as headache, dizziness, digestive upset, tremors, or fatigue haven't disappeared in 5 minutes, drink all the water. Results are often so dramatic, he says, the victim suddenly seems like a new person! Almost 100 percent cures are claimed! If this doesn't work, then allergy is not the cause.

In that case, try nerve massage. One man complained of a terrible headache "the morning after" a drinking party. Nothing he took seemed to bring relief. He was told to rub his thumb (just below the knuckle). He was skeptical but he tried it, and was amazed that his headache was gone almost instantly! The question remains . . .

Why do homeopathic remedies work? The reason, as given by homeopathic doctors, is that a small dose of a homeopathic medicine will give the body a chance to *desensitize* itself to the allergic irritant and produce a buildup of natural substances in the body—in a manner so harmless and painless you don't even notice it. These immunizers *remain* within you for quite some time to neutralize any larger doses of the allergic irritant (like pollen) that may come your way.

Incredible as it may seem, ONE DOSE is all you may need—and symptoms may permanently disappear! Even if the effects are not permanent, says one medical doctor, relief of the symptoms can be continued, which is a blessing for seasonal allergies like hay fever.[5]

In one reported case, Joseph W., 25, a teacher, suffered each spring from acute hay fever that made his life miserable. We are all familiar with how we feel when we peel an onion— the running, burning eyes and nose, the watery and acrid nasal discharge. That's how Joseph W. felt, with constant sneezing and dull headaches which became worse in the evening— especially in a warm room (so that he couldn't relax or concentrate on anything)—but better in fresh air. On advice of

---

[5]James H. Stevenson, M.D. Ibid.

his doctor, he prepared some *Allium cepa* 12x, and is now free of his springtime hay fever!

More Immediate Relief For Hay Fever!

Ms. C.M. writes: "Luckily for me, last summer I (heard about taking) vitamin C, 500 mg. three times daily for hay fever. I have been persecuted for ten years with the curse. I took the vitamins and almost immediately felt better. I could sleep lying down in bed, I could breathe through my nose, my eyes weren't itchy—what a relief!"

A Rose Petal Remedy
For Hay Fever!

In case of hay fever, sore and irritated eyes are reportedly relieved by steeping a few rose petals in a cup of hot water. This is carefully filtered, and the liquid applied to each eye four or five times a day. *Estivin,* a widely-used eyedrop for relief of hay fever, is a "processed infusion of rose petals."

Orange Peels Are Antihistamine!

Mrs. A.R. reports: "I have found orange peel to be the best antihistamine I have ever tried. I have been a victim of allergies all my life. I keep the peels in the refrigerator for several days until there is enough to work up, and I cut them in small strips and soak them in apple cider vinegar solution for several hours, drain off well, place in pan with honey and cook them down, but not to the candy stage. Then I put them in the refrigerator and eat as I need them. I place some pieces in my mouth when I go to bed at night. No more stuffiness and clogged air passages to keep waking me from sleep."

Tangerine For Runny Nose!

Mr. G.E. reports: "In this smog-infested city, I have trouble at night with a runny nose. It lasts for 2 to 3 hours. I decided to try tangerine peel, having heard that they are highest in bioflavonoids. It works! Stops running nose within five to ten minutes. I dry the peel at room temperature for a week, break off a piece, approximately one inch square, chew and swallow it."

Allergies, Asthma, and Nasal Polyps Relieved!

Mrs. S.W. reports: "Now, after two years of good health and comfort following 16 years of suffering with allergies, asthma and nasal polyps, I feel the urge to share my findings.

"**Medications, allergy tests, shots, fasts, diets, inhalants, heart cardiograms, blood tests, hypoglycemia tests, oxygen masks, temperature and pulse charts, extra dental work and seven nose operations for the removal of over 130 polyps still left me utterly miserable and short $25,000 which I had spent.**

"Then someone told me about rutin as an aid to allergies, as well as natural vitamins and minerals. Every day I take vitamin A, brewer's yeast, B multiple (heavy potency), 1,000 to 1,500 mg. vitamin C with bioflavonoids and rutin, 50 mg. extra rutin, 400 units of vitamin D, 600 I.U. vitamin E, three unsaturated fatty acid capsules, three lecithin capsules, six bone meal, two garlic perles and six sea kelp.

"The results are worth shouting about. I am 56 years old, work nine hours a day, manage and keep up a large home, do some entertaining and have time to sew all my own clothes. I have come back from a gasping, wheezing individual with my nose grown shut with polyps to one with endless enthusiasm and strength!"

11

Miracles Medicine Foods For The Nerves!

One doctor claimed that taking a little apple cider vinegar in water daily, or two teaspoons of honey, will stop any headache—even a migraine—within a half hour. Another method he recommended was to place equal parts of apple cider vinegar in water in a steamer, cover your head with a towel and inhale 75 breaths. This, too, was supposed to relieve the headache in a half hour!

A woman who suffered migraine headaches reports that she cures them by taking a tablespoon of honey, as soon as she feels one coming on. If the headache returns, she follows with a second dose of honey and three glasses of water. Her headache disappears completely and doesn't return.

Mr. S.W. writes: "Since ten years of age I have had migraine headaches—very severe at times, putting me in bed for two or three days. . . . Last summer I had a large garden on a vacant lot next to my home and grew lots of vegetables and we had fruit. . . . I had no headaches from July until Thanksgiving. Then the headaches came again, after the garden produce gave out, for I ate them lusciously—tomatoes, cabbage, cucumbers, radishes, etc., with the raw fruit from our yard.

"I concluded that my system needed these raw vegetables for enzymes, minerals and bulk. I began eating these things with every meal, and behold, my migraine headaches stopped. Twice a day I drink strong herb teas, not straining them, but also eating the grinds. I am 78 years old.... After all these years, I am so happy to know how to stop migraine headaches."

Lecithin For Migraine!

Mrs. A.M. reports: "I cured my migraine headaches with lecithin. For around six years I've been plagued by migraines and wouldn't go anywhere without my bottle of Fiorinal. Then some months ago I remembered an old man telling me that if he didn't take lecithin he couldn't control his temper.

> "I'm an extremely nervous person, so I figured if it could help his temper it could probably help my nerves. When I started taking lecithin I would still get headaches (though much milder) and instead of taking Fiorinal I would take an extra dosage of lecithin right when the headache started and it worked."

Mrs. A.V. reports: "I have suffered from migraine since I was nine years old (I am now 36). I have been taking lecithin regularly, and increase the amount when I feel I have a headache coming on. *I have not taken one Fiorinal tablet since that time*. I am most grateful and thankful for this, as anyone who has ever experienced migraine headaches could certainly appreciate."

Other Remedies For Migraine!

Mrs. S.R. reports: "I have been plagued with migraine-type headaches as long as I can remember. I awaken at 3 to 4 a.m. three or four times weekly. I have tried any suggestion anyone offered.

> "Last year I increased my brewer's yeast to nine tablets daily, and since the first week (nearly 10 months ago) I am completely relieved of headaches. I can't tell you what a relief it is, after all these years (I'm 54)!"

Yet another woman, 26, suffering with migraines since age 15, started taking vitamins C, E, B complex, calcium and iron daily and twice as much during her periods. She says: "I truly believe that taking these vitamins has changed my life. There's no more suffering with migraines for me!"[1]

Within An Hour ... Depression Vanished!

Mr. A.N. reports: "Last August I had a sudden attack of acute schizophrenia and was hospitalized for three months. When I left the hospital, I was 30 pounds overweight, rundown, depressed and fearful. Since I received no help or advice, I decided to do my own research, and learned of vitamin B-3 treatment for schizophrenics. I stocked up on a niacinamide (B-3) and other vitamins and began self-treatment.

"Within an hour after taking massive doses of niacinamide my depression vanished not to return. In a month I had a complete personality change. Self-confidence returned, fear left, I became vibrant, alert, energetic. Friends were amazed. Niacinamide is also used in treating alcoholism."

Tingling Hands Are Pain-Free and Stronger Than Ever!

Mr. A.R. reports: "I suffered from weak, tingling hands for over a year. I couldn't even hold a razor in my hand to shave myself. If I brushed my fingers against an object the pain was extreme. I had to sleep with a pail of water filled with ice cubes alongside my bed. In the event I awakened because of the pain I would plunge my hand, either left or right, into the pail of ice water to numb it.

---

[1] Eat all the spinach you can, says medical experts. It's loaded with an enzyme which breaks down headache-causing chemicals called amines. Avoid all smoked, pickled or fermented foods, alcohol, chocolate, cheeses, milk, bananas and citrus. Cut down on fatty fried foods, coffee, tea and sea foods, say these doctors. Eliminating food containing monosodium glutamate, and not skipping meals (which causes low blood sugar) can relieve migraines! Well balanced meals are recommended.

"I consulted six orthopedic doctors. They all concluded that my problem was carpal tunnel syndrome. Finally, finding it impossible to work and unable to stand the pain, I agreed to have the surgery performed. The night before the operation, I lay in my hospital bed wide awake until midnight when I asked the nurse for a sleeping pill. She refused. So I told her I was going home. She laughed and said, 'You wouldn't.' Well, she wouldn't and I did. I ducked down the stairs and out of the hospital.

"The following week I consulted another doctor, a nutritionist. I described my symptoms and she prescribed vitamin B-6, 200 mg. three times a day. It took exactly six weeks for the symptoms to clear up. My hands are pain-free and stronger than ever."

Trembling Quickly Relieved!

Mrs. T.J. reports: "Six months ago I began to shake, especially in the legs, and elsewhere. My doctor said it was nerves and possibly the beginning of Parkinson's disease. A registered nurse told me people on high blood pressure medication will shake and tremble because the medication destroys potassium. My doctor finally gave me a prescription for potassium and the improvement was noticeable within three days! Why didn't he think of that? I am practically free of the shaking now." (Potassium tablets are available at health stores, without prescription.)

Miracle Medicine Foods
For Neuritis and Sciatica!

Sciatica is a painful inflammation of the sciatic nerve which runs down the back of the thigh and leg. Dr. E. Braner, reporting in the *British Medical Journal* (April 15, 1944), tells of relieving this condition quickly with injections of vitamin B-1. Eating garlic along with vitamin B-1 gives the same effect as injections, according to the Japanese scientist Fujiwara, as reported in the *Pakistan Medical Times* (May 16, 1961). Foods rich in B-1 include lean pork, beans, dried peas, nuts, liver, other meats, milk and eggs.

Spasms of the face, with pain of a stabbing or throbbing nature, and twitching, is known as tic douloureux or trigeminal neuralgia. Many drugs have been used to treat this condition. Surgery may relieve it. In 1914, a Prague doctor cured 48 cases with pure elderberry juice!

Patients took 20 grams daily for five days. Some were cured with only one dose! Others after a few days. It was discovered that adding 20% alcohol speeded the healing. Two years later a Norwegian doctor combined 10 grams of port wine with 30 grams of elderberry juice, and discovered that acute cases of sciatica were cured in as little as one day! No case lasted longer than two or three weeks.

Painful Sciatica Relieved By Miracle Medicine Foods!

Mrs. A.N. reports: "I had a case of sciatica that was almost unbearable. Every kind of test and x-ray was used but no direct cause was found. Traction was applied with no relief. The doctors decided to give me large doses of protein (in gelatin form) as well as shots of vitamin B-12. When the pain finally subsided, my left leg was almost useless. I had to learn to walk all over again. That was 3½ years ago, after a five-week siege in the hospital. A short time later, I began taking a vitamin supplement plus vitamin E, bone meal, dessicated liver tablets, brewer's yeast, and lots of vitamin C all day long.

"I haven't had a cold in three years. No aches or pains, and I work 8 hours a day as a seamstress. Everyone wants to know where I get all my energy. However, few really believe me when I tell them!"

Leg Cramp Relieved!

Mr. R.G. reports: "I found that by wearing warm clothing in bed and not getting cold I could prevent my terrible leg cramps. Then about eight months ago I started taking daily 200 units of vitamin E, 500 mg. of vitamin C, one dolomite tablet containing bone meal, liver and yeast. What happened? A miracle! No longer do I have to wear warm things in bed, in fact, I wear nothing on my legs. Only those who have suffered these terrible cramps can appreciate the wonderful relief!

"As a side effect, my hair is turning dark! (I am 85.) My wife first noticed it and now others have also noticed it."

Herpes Zoster (Shingles) Relieved!

Dr. A.L. Oriz relieved the painful clustering of small blisters, known as "shingles" or *herpes zoster*, in 25 cases, with intra-muscular injections of thiamin hydrochloride, according to *Medical World News* (November 1958). Other doctors have achieved the same results. Thiamin is vitamin B-1.

Mrs. S.C. reports: "Many years ago I had shingles on my left thigh. The doctor said it was inflammation of the nerve ends but gave no medicine. At home I reasoned: nerves need vitamin B, the best source is liver. A week later the doctor asked, 'Is it very painful?' He was surprised when I said no. I take dessicated liver. The taste is strong so I put it in milk and blackstrap molasses, one-half cup milk, two tablespoons molasses, one-half teaspoon liver. Let it set a while and the liver grains soften...." Her shingles hasn't bothered her in years.

Miracle Medicine Foods Heal
Horrible Case of Shingles!

A.N. reports: "A couple of years ago I showed my chest to my M.D. and he gravely informed me that I had a severe form of shingles. They were all around my back and my chest and refused to be ignored. They'd run you wild. I promptly stocked up on high concentrations of the B vitamins as well as all other vitamins, especially E and a big bottle of E liquid —the oil to be applied liberally over all red spots on my chest and back. Two weeks later I kept my appointment with the doctor and cheerfully removed my shirt. He gaped in utter amazement and disbelief. He said, 'I *never* saw anything like that before! What in heaven's name did you put on it?' When I told him vitamin E oil, he sneered. Needless to say, I soon healed up."

Immediate Relief for Shingles!

Another woman, Mrs. L.V. says she got instant relief from shingles with a common herb—goldenseal—available at most health stores in powder or capsule form. She dissolved some in water, and applied it to the area several times a day and before bed. This worked after a doctor's lotion failed. "Almost immediately," she says, "the shingles started drying up." In two weeks, it was completely gone. She also drank one capsule with warm water an hour before each meal (reportedly, a safer dose is 1/3 teaspoon daily, no more).

The Miracle Medicine Food That Cured the Incurable!

Multiple sclerosis has been repeatedly cured in lab animals by adding manganese to their food, according to Dr. Robert Hill, of the Mercy Institute for Biomedical Research. Step one was to feed the animals only milk—which lacks manganese. Even though the milk was fortified with vitamins, Dr. Hill was able to cause a breakdown in the myelin sheath —the nerve protector—in these animals. (This breakdown is the acknowledged cause of MS).

The symptoms of multiple sclerosis could be *reversed* by adding manganese sulfate to the diet of the animals, according to a report on Dr. Hill's work in the *Denver Post,* August 13, 1974. In work sponsored by the Public Health Service in 1958, other doctors obtained the same results!

The Miracle Medicine Food That Halted MS!

In one reported case, a young M.D. was able to halt the progress of his own MS by eating buckwheat cakes—on the advise of Dr. Hill. Buckwheat is rich in manganese. He quickly saw his symptoms (muscle jerking, tremors, and lack of coordination) disappear, and they have never returned. Yet we are constantly told MS is incurable!

Another Miracle Medicine
Food Halts MS!

Miss L.A. writes: "I was diagnosed as having MS in April, 1975 by (two doctors). My whole left side was weak and my left leg was so stiff that at times I could not go up and down the stairs. I was taking every kind of vitamin supplement there is but that didn't seem to improve me. Around the first of June I remembered a book I had read ... written by an M.D. ... He said vinegar builds strong muscles. I started drinking about one ounce a day mixed with honey.

"About a week later, I went to see my doctor and my feet did not tremble any more. He said I was definitely better. I was still weak though so I started drinking a half glass a day. The improvement was dramatic. I have most of my strength back now ... I don't know why, but vinegar has helped me more than anything else ..."

A Biochemist Heals Himself!

A biochemist reporting in *Lancet,* October 15, 1970, states: "Five years ago, I was told I had multiple sclerosis. From the diagnosis in 1969 until early 1973 I became slowly worse ... I felt apathetic, I tired easily. I had backaches, my balance was bad, I had flickering in my eyes, and one hand was numb and sensory paralysis was creeping up my arm."

In March 1973, he began taking a number of vitamins and minerals, including 900 mg. of magnesium daily—and reduced his white sugar intake, avoiding bread products. He says: "In two months, I felt more alert and a few months later the flickering in my eyes and the backache had gone (just some numbness in fingers remained)." He found he could take magnesium alone—and no other supplements—with continued improvement.

After 20 Years Multiple Sclerosis Gone!

Mrs. G.T. reports: "I have had multiple sclerosis for over 20 years, with many relapses and remissions. But for the past 18 years since I began my diet (and quit smoking) I have had no further trouble.

"I was hit hard when I was taken to Mayo Clinic and told, after a spinal tap, that I had multiple sclerosis and nothing could be done. It was incurable. I was so depressed that in a few days I was much worse off than when I first came to the hospital. I literally had no leg to stand on and only with great effort could walk in a very grotesque manner, swinging my right leg way out to the right.

"Yes, I was numb over most of my body, especially my arms and legs. It was not long before I was having extreme difficulty swallowing my food. . . . A little later I also became incontinent (couldn't hold my urine), which lasted a long time until I accidentally discovered that magnesium in the form of dolomite powder could control it. This happened in only one day and was a most blessed relief. Yes, I could talk a 'blue streak' about the wonders of good nutrition and the fact of it having brought me back from what looked like a really hopeless condition. For eight years I have eaten no refined flour in any form. I have experienced this reversal in spite of a broken hip shattered by a purse snatcher. If I can do it, surely there must be hope for others, working with a nutritionally oriented physician!"

Nerve-Caused Blindness Cured!

Mr. M.P. writes: "Eight years ago I had a neurological problem which was diagnosed as a 'degenerative neurological disorder symptomatic of MS'—I spent three weeks in the hospital and was given 80 units of ACTH a day for twelve days as treatment. I was unable to work for almost a year and had a lot of time to do a lot of research on my own.

"I concluded that possibly the intake of linoleic acid and

polyunsaturated fat might have something to do with this type of illness. Consequently I put myself on a diet high in polyunsaturates which I felt would be high in linoleic acid. This included safflower oil, sunflower seeds,[2] vitamin E and a host of other supplements.

"I was blind in my left eye, my coordination and speech were affected, and I was numb in various parts of my body. However, my sight has returned and all the symptoms have disappeared with no relapse.

"I am still on my diet and safflower oil, and my local physician tells me to keep on doing whatever I have been doing. I had been on medication for leg cramps but am no longer on it."

Myasthenia Gravis Disappears!

Myasthenia gravis has been cured in patients given a diet high in protein, vitamin E, all the B vitamins, and manganese, according to Dr. Emannuel Josephson in his book, *The Thymus, Manganese and Myasthenia Gravis* (Chedney Press, 1961). Relief was prompt. All the classical symptoms and other forms of paralysis disappeared within a few weeks. The results were said to have been "rapid and astonishing!" Yet every day—on TV and the mass media—we are told this ailment is incurable!

Miracle Medicine Food
Relieves Muscular Dystrophy!

We are told that 25 children afflicted with the crippling and wasting disease known as muscular dystrophy were given wheat germ oil daily,[3] plus vitamins C and B. Every child im-

---

[2]Multiple sclerosis, deemed incurable, has been greatly relieved by taking 2 tablespoons of sunflower seed oil twice a day, according to Dr. Harold Miller and associates at the Royal Victoria Hospital, Belfast, Northern Ireland (*British Medical Journal*, March 31, 1973). It seems to prolong quiescent periods.

[3]"Experiments with Wheat Germ Oil," *Journal of Neurology, Neurosurgery and Psychiatry* (London, May 1951).

proved under this plan, and there was one complete recovery. In another experiment, 151 patients with various nerve-muscle disorders were given wheat germ oil. Their progress was followed for twelve years:

- **In five (three children and two adults) out of 25 patients with progressive muscular dystrophy, symptoms were arrested and moderate to marked improvement occurred.**
- **Three out of five patients with menopausal muscular dystrophy showed remarkable improvement. (Other than the wheat germ oil, these patients were not placed on any particular diet.)**

Cerebral Palsy Healed!

A 7-year-old boy, Tommy, was suffering from cerebral palsy, which caused spastic paralysis of his arms and legs (wild, jerky movements) and affected his speech. The doctor shook his head: no cure for cerebral palsy. Tommy was due to be fitted for a back brace to support his withered muscles.

Meanwhile, someone suggested a Miracle Medicine Food —wheat germ oil—which has been shown to bring relief in cases of cerebral palsy. Other Miracle Medicine Foods were added including proteins, vitamins and minerals. A month later, when Tommy came in for his brace, it didn't fit! His withered muscles had firmed up!

Later, a snapshot of Tommy was sent to the doctor to show his amazing progress. The photo showed the boy whizzing by on a bicycle, for he was so healthy he could run and play like any normal child! Yet every day, on TV, we are told that cerebral palsy is incurable!

Hopelessly Paralyzed Girl Cured With Sunflower Seed Oil!

In a recently reported case, sunflower seed oil was used to cure Lydia, a seven-year-old girl who was hopelessly paralyzed by a virus that attacked her nervous system. The virus, known as polyneuritis, causes white blood cells to stop doing their job, which is to fight viruses. Instead, they attack healthy nerve tissue. In three weeks, the little girl was almost totally paralyzed and could not move her arms or legs. She'd wake up screaming—terrified because she couldn't move. Doctors said she would remain permanently paralyzed for life.

Then her parents heard a doctor on TV tell of amazing results he had obtained by giving sunflower oil to kidney transplant patients—preventing white blood cells from attacking and rejecting the new kidney. So they bought a bottle of ordinary sunflower oil from a local health food store, and gave her a teaspoonful three times a day. Miraculously, in 48 hours, she began to move! Her father doubled the dosage, and she continued to improve. Soon she could run and jump and play, like any other little girl her age, and today she seems completely normal!

Dolomite Fights Epilepsy!

Mrs. J.J. reports: "I've been taking magnesium to control my epilepsy now for 18 months. I am 50 years old and have suffered with this illness since I was 17 years old. I went to doctors, and had EEG tests without results. I tried several drugs and at last had my seizures reduced by one of them. But I still was always tense and nervous, and lived with constant fear of the next attack. My physician was not helpful.

"Then I heard about magnesium, started taking two dolomite tablets a day, with my regular medication, and I have not had one petit mal or grand mal attack in 18 months. I hope others who have suffered may try this. I also take brewer's yeast, dessicated liver, vitamin C and E for circulation and dolomite.

"I was a walking corpse before I started this program. Now I work every day as a nurse's aide, and am just starting to live my next fifty years." (Note: apropos of the two preceding cases, it has been found that vitamin B-6, *pyridoxine*, can control polyneuritis and epilepsy.)

Epilepsy, Paralysis, and Blindness Miraculously Treated!

In *Summary* (June 1961), Dr. Alfonso del Guidice, of the National Institute of Public Health, Buenos Aires, Argentina says that in cases of nerve-caused eye ailments treated with vitamin E, he has had "brilliant results" with myopia (nearsightedness), nystogmus (involuntary rapid eye movements), strabismus (crossed eyes), cataract, paralysis and epilepsy. Every patient improved!

"Generally we have begun treatment with 200 or 300 milligrams of vitamin E daily, increasing over a period of as long as 6 months, doses approximating two grams daily," depending on the age of the patient. "Vitamin C was also given in doses of 500 to 1500 mg. daily. It was added because of my belief that it reinforces vitamin E (and) seems especially indicated in organic deficiencies and old cataracts." But for these patients, vitamin E was the miracle medicine food, he emphasizes. Relief seemed permanent.

Reported Cases:

- A girl, 3, was suffering from epilepsy (resulting from a bad fall). At the age of 2, she had her first seizure, lasting four minutes, with unconsciousness, spasm and frothing at the mouth, followed by a violent headache lasting six hours. For ninety minutes she was unable to speak. After that, she was nervous, restless, had crying spells and wet the bed. Vitamin E was started as the only treatment. In three months she had no more convulsions, and in less than a year she stopped her bed-wetting and became friendly and normal.
- A 9-month-old boy was diagnosed as epileptic. He had convulsions several times daily during which his eyes pulled to one side, his neck became rigid, and he lost consciousness. He was nervous and restless. Drugs and sedatives did not help. Then he was given vitamin E only. In five months, he had no more convlusions and slept peacefully!
- A girl, 12, was mentally retarded and violent. She

shouted and cried all the time, was unable to speak properly, could not understand questions or manage her toilet functions. This had been going on six years. No treatment helped. In a little over a month on vitamin E, she suddenly improved, became quiet, sat correctly and ate by herself by the end of the year.
- A girl, 5 was paralyzed in both legs, and retarded. She could not speak. All treatments had failed, since birth. After seven months on vitamin E she began to walk and talk clearly. Four months later, she could even run!
- A man, 23, suffered nerve-caused blindness. His eyes were normal, but he could not see. Eight years of treatment had failed. In less than 2 months on vitamin E, he could see the fingers on a hand almost seven feet away, and recognize people ten feet away, with his left eye. With his right eye he saw a little less, but he could now dress and feed himself, travel alone and walk through city traffic!
- A girl, 10, born with cataracts on both eyes, was totally blind. She could not see light, even after an operation on her right eye. She was extremely quiet and depressed. After six months of vitamin E, she became cheerful, and could see light! The cataracts were disappearing. Her right eyeball was now clearly visible!
- A boy, 10, born with cataracts on one eye and defects in both eyes, was also retarded. Vitamin E therapy was begun. He became brighter and more alert, the cataracts disappeared, and vision in both eyes improved. All this started immediately.
- A child, 10, born with cataracts on both eyes (both operated on unsuccessfully), started taking vitamin E. In eight months, she could see small objects at a distance!

The Blind Can Now See— And The Deaf Can Now Hear!

"I want to tell you the great news that the blind can now see and the deaf can now hear," says Reginald MacNitt,

Ph.D., in his book, *How to Use Astral Power* (Parker Publishing Company, Inc., 1977). "Restored hearing and vision are among the minor miracles produced by Astral Power," says Dr. MacNitt, referring to extrasensory sight and sound, which has, in fact, been used by totally blind and deaf people to see and hear.

"Yes, it is true," he emphasizes, referring to seemingly hopeless cases. "Every blind and deaf person in the world can experience these things," he says. "They will not be blind, deaf or crippled. They can see, hear or experience any of the many wonderful sensations, with the miracle of Astral Power!"

"If you are blind, or deaf," says Dr. MacNitt, "this secret will make it possible for you to hear your own voice. You can look at television. You can enter into conversation and see all of your friends around you. You can hear and see the world as it really is. As a blind person, you will no longer need to go around feeling faces and objects. You will know what others look like." If you are deaf, "you will no longer need to learn sign language..." Other researchers claim—

Eyeless Sight!

If, for example, every other means of transmitting visual images to the brain were destroyed, it could still receive them through its visual control center. The brain itself has billions of microscopic "hair" cells, extremely sensitive to all electrical impressions around them. Thus, we have numerous cases on record of people who have been able to see out of the back or top of their heads. The famous German researcher, Dr. Albert von Schrenck-Notzing reported in 1887 how a subject named Lina was able to read books, while blindfolded, in this manner. Experts say anyone can do it, with patient mindpower training.

The most famous case of this kind was Mollie Fancher, blinded after a serious accident that destroyed her eyes. And yet she could see as clearly as any normal person—

clearer, in fact. She could see through her forehead. She knew what was going on around her, and could describe the minutest movements of any visitor. She clearly saw colors, and could knit and crochet! She could read in light or darkness—much more rapidly than you or I —by running her fingers over the printed page!

Scientists have long known that the entire epidermis or outer skin covering the body contains photoelectric cells that can transmit actual seeing impressions to the brain. Cesare Lombroso, the world-famous psychologist, and Professor Carmagnola, reported two such cases in the *Italian Medical Journal*. Both girls, age 14, were quite blind but saw as clearly as before—one with the tip of her nose. The other could see easily with the palms of her hands. In both cases, the girls could read any printed matter selected at random.

Any Form Of Blindness Or Deafness Can Be Cured, Say Experts, With This Secret!

Both the sight and hearing centers of the brain remain receptive to any impressions that can get through, say mind power experts—even if the eyes and ears are destroyed. Reportedly, one method of developing extrasensory sight and hearing is to induce a light self-hypnotic trance by concentrating on one thing. When you are in a dream-like reverie, focus your mind on any impressions you wish to receive. It is now that your Third Eye—or mind's eye—may be focused on that which you wish to see or hear. With tactile sensations through the hands it is also a guessing game that requires persistent practice and a positive mental attitude in the face of all evidence to the contrary.

But Dr. MacNitt's method goes beyond extra-sensory perception and includes actual healing of diseased organs, in some cases.[4] For a more detailed account of how his

---

[4] In his book, *How to Use Astral Power*, Dr. MacNitt tells how a patient named Charlotte noticed that she could not see clearly.

method works see pages 40 to 44. Many experts agree this is possible.

Among these experts is Evelyn Monahan, whose much-acclaimed course at the University of Georgia's School of Adult Education was widely reported in *Time, Newsweek, Midnight* and the *National Enquirer*. For five years, she taught blind people to see with their hands, and many obtained skilled jobs, like reading blueprints! She also says that mind power can heal diseased organs.

Blindness, Paralysis and Epilepsy Cured In Ten Days!

In her book, *The Miracle of Metaphysical Healing* (Parker Publishing Company, Inc., 1975), Dr. Monohan tells how she was *cured* of these three incurable ailments—after 9 years of suffering—instantly and spontaneously in 10 days, with mind power. As a result of an accident, her vision had been reduced to a pinhole and was fading, and she experienced epileptic seizures (as many as 12 a day even with drugs). Two years later, she suffered another serious accident, which left her right arm paralyzed. Imagine it! Blind, paralyzed and epileptic! Eleven medical specialists said her paralysis was hopeless.

The method she used to heal her blinded, paralyzed, and spasmodic nerves was mind power, which she says can even be used to heal others, at a distance, and is even more powerful if more than one person concentrates on it, using the same method. The method is essentially strong visualization and positive thinking, with affirmation that you *are being* cured (not "will" or "may"), with doctors and friends congratulating you on that fact—completely blotting out any negative thoughts, several times a day.

An eye specialist told her that she had a cataract and needed an operation. With this amazing method, her cataract disappeared in one day like magic, and the vision in both her eyes was restored to nearly perfect 20/20!

In describing her method, Dr. Monohan calls it a "cure" and says it is the exact one she followed to bring a healing to herself, and receive a complete cure from blindness. "With this method," she says, "you will find that a healing is not long in coming, bringing its gift of eyesight to the person for whom it is used." In addition, she says. "This miraculous technique is guaranteed to bring the blessing of perfect health to you and any of your loved ones who suffer from epilepsy." And she adds that this method worked for her and countless others in restoring freedom of movement to paralyzed limbs. She says it will bring miracle healing to anyone suffering "any form of paralysis." She says it is guaranteed to work, and cannot fail. If mind power can heal the nerves, then it is obviously miracle medicine food for the nerves.

Reported Cases:
- David L., 19, awoke one morning totally paralyzed from the neck down. He could only move his eyes and lips. Doctors were baffled, as they could find no reason for his paralysis. A champion athlete, he spent the next five-and-a-half years flat on his back, staring at the ceiling. Then Dr. Monahan showed David and his mother how this method works. Within two-and-a-half weeks he was completely cured, able to move freely!
- John's right arm had been paralyzed for three years following an accident in which several nerves had been severed. John did not believe this method would work for him, and was full of anger and resentment at being crippled. Yet when Dr. Monahan explained how her own paralysis had been cured, he agreed to it. Within two weeks, his paralysis was completely gone, and you would never guess that he had ever been paralyzed!

Hundreds Report Miraculous Cures With Medipic!

Hundreds report miraculous cures of seemingly hopeless ailments, with Medipic, a seventh-sense healing method, according to Benjamin O. Bibb and Joseph J. Weed in *Amazing Secrets of Psychic Healing* (Parker Publishing Company, Inc.,

1976). "Actually," say Bibb and Weed, "every human malfunction can be corrected" with this secret! Even in terminal cases, you can often buy extra time! If the inner mind can be convinced of it, they add, "No healing is impossible!"

> How often have you heard there is no cure for the common cold? But there is—say Bibb and Weed—"the subject's inner mind can cure it, often within minutes." By simply thinking on it, you can suggest telepathically to the inner mind a way to do this.

Use clear mental pictures of the things you want done. That is the way to communicate with the inner mind. For example, if there is some obstruction, visualize healing fingers gently lifting it away and removing it. "Mental fingers," a "mental brush or pipe cleaner," or "mental adhesive tape" may sound like silly imaginary things, but they are the kind of clear mental pictures your inner mind needs if you are to communicate with it and tell it what to do. Having told your inner mind the steps it needs to take to relieve an ailment, *it will find a way* to make these things happen inside your body, for the mind can control the body. It can control all the functions NORMALLY controlled by the central nervous system. It can take control, something like when a machine that is programmed to operate automatically is switched to "manual"—so that a human can make it do something it doesn't normally do.

Amazing Results Claimed!
- In cases of nearsightedness or farsightedness, say Bibb and Weed, "Whatever the cause . . . you can in almost every case either remedy or cure both these afflictions and astigmatism (eye imbalance)." Eye muscles can be strengthened, mentally, in 24 hours!
- You can "permanently correct or cure glaucoma" with this method, say Bibb and Weed. "Regardless of the cause you can relieve glaucoma quickly and easily"—although it will not remain so unless nervous tension is permanently avoided. "In almost every case" they say,

"this will restore the (eye) to its normal function and relieve the ... tension and pain of glaucoma."
- When the liver is causing pain this method is the simplest and best treatment—and will also help cirrhosis, jaundice, hepatitis and fibrosis of the liver—say Bibb and Weed: "Very often this will be the only remedy required (and) will relieve the sufferer completely," say Bibb and Weed.
- Gallstones are relieved the same way. "Mentally, you can dissolve and remove all stones from the gall bladder," say Bibb and Weed: "We have demonstrated complete and often what appears to be permanent relief of this condition," without surgery!
- All forms of intestinal upset can be helped easily with this method, say Bibb and Weed—including appendicitis, gastroenteritis, diverticulitis, intestinal obstruction, ulcers, dysentery or food poisoning. Ulcers are fused shut! Diverticuli sacs are removed from the intestinal wall!
- Medipic can stop arthritis pain, and frequently cure it, say Bibb and Weed. "Rapid relief can be afforded a bursitis sufferer ... The mind can cure tendonitis. ... Like bursitis, it can be cleared up quickly, usually within an hour or so," they state. Calcium deposits are removed and joints are lubricated!
- "In all cases of spinal damage or breakdown (including fibromyositis, tenderness, pain and stiffness of joints and muscles, lumbago, shoulder pain, thigh pain or charley horse) ... *Each of these ailments may be cured* by the Medipic method," say Bibb and Weed. Ruptured discs and even spinal birth deformities—deemed incurable by doctors—can be healed, they add. Osteomyelitis (a type of bone infection) can be treated successfully this way, and bone tumors and tuberculosis of the bones and joints can be removed, say Bibb and Weed.
- Damaged veins and arteries (including varicose veins) and blood problems ranging from anemia to blood poisoning, hemorrhage and dangerous blood clots "can

all be healed by Medipic treatments," say Bibb and Weed.
- Leukemia ("invariably fatal" in 6 to 12 months, according to Stedman's Medical Dictionary) can be cured, say Bibb and Weed. Their method, they say, restores normal red-white blood cell balance and clears the system of accumulated debris "in almost all cases" and "may be employed to effect a cure."
- Hemophilia, the bleeding disease, deemed incurable, "can be corrected by Medipic methods" by stimulating the blood to produce coagulants, say Bibb and Weed.
- Hodgkin's disease ("usually fatal in five years") can be helped by Medipic, say the authors. "In many cases this will achieve relief and accomplish a cure."

Medipic can "relieve pain in a matter of minutes," say Bibb and Weed. It can "heal wounds, cuts and abrasions *the day they are suffered*"—and they cite cases of serious burns, large open cuts, and wounds virtually healing over before the astonished victim's eyes, leaving only a tiny smooth red spot that also fades. This method can "strengthen the heart and repair any malfunctions that hamper its action," "heal diabetes," bring "instantaneous" prostate relief, and much more.

It is hard to dismiss these astonishing claims in light of the proof given. Bibb and Weed quote actual letters from people who achieved these amazing results.

Reported Cases:
- A woman had a painful blood clot in her leg, with blue marks on it. Her doctor said she needed an operation. She was frightened. With this method, the next morning the clot had liquefied and disappeared. Her doctor found no trace of it and was amazed!
- A boy was nearly blinded by a detached lens. With this method, the lens was "glued" back in place the next day. Doctors were amazed. It looked solid. He now has 20/20 vision and is completely cured!
- A man was suffering from leukemia, and had been receiving "packed" transfusions for a long time. With

this method, in three weeks his red blood count was normal and he never needed blood transfusions again. His doctors were flabbergasted.
- A woman was so sick with a liver ailment she could not hold any food and had cramps and nausea for a week. A doctor's medication did not help. With this method, she felt so good she ate a delicious meal and kept the whole thing down, and was never bothered again!
- A man with gallstones was awakened at 2 a.m. with excruciating chest pain and nausea. He thought it was a heart attack and threw up several times. With this method, in a few minutes he fell asleep and awoke the next morning with no pain.
- A man was flat on his back, in agony, with a ruptured disc. Drugs gave no relief. With this method, all pain disappeared in a few days, and did not return. He is now back at work in a job requiring a lot of bending, lifting and crawling, and feels fine.
- A woman had a tumor the size of an egg in her rectum, near her uterus. Her doctor advised immediate surgery. She was constipated, with bloody stools, her Pap test and X-rays were positive, and she was very frightened. With this method, the tumor slowly disappeared, and doctors now found it was harmless!

If Astral Power, Metaphysical Healing, Positive Thinking, Meditation Therapy, Medipic or any other mind power method can do this, clearly it is miracle medicine food for the body. It seems perfectly safe to use along with—not as a substitute for—qualified medical care!

12

Miracle Medicine Foods For Women's Problems!

Miss B.R. reports: "I am a 26-year-old woman and for many years had painful and heavy menstrual periods. Two and sometimes three aspirins did not relieve the pain, so I would take four to five aspirins within two to three hours until the pain was relieved.

"The bleeding was almost hemorrhagic, and I finally realized it had something to do with the aspirin. Last month I took two dolomite tablets instead of aspirin. Within 20 minutes the menstrual pains were gone and the menstrual blood loss was minimal. I genuinely believe this saved me from chronic anemia."

Dolomite, of course, contains calcium and magnesium. What is it that makes calcium so important to a woman's body? Scientists tell us that poor diet plus a drastic calcium loss during menstruation play havoc with a woman's body.

Breast Pain Vanished Immediately!

Ms. H.L. reports: "For about four years now I have suffered with very painful breasts, ten days to two weeks before each period. I was so sore I couldn't sleep on my stomach. Then I began taking bone meal and dolomite tablets, which I bought at a health food store.

"I suddenly noticed I was not having all this pain anymore, and told a co-worker who had the same problems that it must be the bone meal and dolomite tablets. She started taking them and also found great relief.

"This summer while on vacation I didn't take them and all I can say is that I was sorry. That month the pain was as bad as before. I had almost forgotten how bad it could be. I have been taking them regularly now, and what a blessing."

Instant Pain Relief for Menstrual Cramps!

Thus, we see how important calcium is to a woman. Increased calcium intake can do a lot to relieve menstrual and menopausal problems.

Reportedly, calcium can relieve both premenstrual tension and menstrual cramps. Menstrual cramps usually disappear within half an hour after calcium is taken. Even during menopause, when calcium is taken, hot flashes, night sweats, leg cramps, and mental depression will often disappear, say experts.

Even birth pains are reduced to the point where some mothers have claimed their delivery was entirely painless—just like mild "gas" sensations! Foods rich in calcium include common beans, beet greens, chard, watercress, dandelion greens, endive, kale, mustard greens, parsley, turnip greens, milk and eggs.

How This Secret Relieved Her Menstrual Pain!

Mrs. R.L. reports: "Calcium has set me completely free of drugs. I double or triple my daily intake of calcium as soon as I feel the tension mounting the day before my period starts. When cramps are anticipated, I take still more calcium (always being sure to get adequate amounts of magnesium, vitamin D and oil for fat). As a matter of fact, when both my babies were born, calcium was my only pain reliever. It worked beautifully."

One woman writes: "My 15-year-old daughter has suffered menstrual cramps since the age of 11. Then she began taking bone meal with vitamin D immediately upon sight of her period, and now she does not know what it is to have cramps. I thought you'd like to know about this cure."

Other Foods Relieve Menstrual Problems!

Practically every ache and pain a woman experiences can be traced to poor diet plus a loss of vital nutrients, such as iron (for oxygen and energy), B complex and copper (for the nerves and for iron absorption), potassium (which relieves swelling and keeps muscles from cramping), magnesium (the mineral that keeps skin smooth and works with the B complex to control the nerves of coordination), vitamins C and D (for resistance to infection)—all these are at a low level during menstruation due to blood loss and hormone imbalance. That is why certain foods rich in vital nutrients can bring relief from menstrual problems.

Swollen Hands and Feet Relieved Quickly!

One doctor reports that vitamin B-6 relieves swelling and water retention, and seemed to work where diuretics failed. One woman suffered puffy hands and fingers so painful she could hardly lift anything—diagnosed as premenstrual water retention (edema). He prescribed two 50 mg. tablets of B-6 daily. In three days she could wear her rings, type, and had no pain or swelling. She now takes one tablet daily, 10 days before her period. A woman eight months pregnant with extremely swollen feet was given 50 mg. injections of B-6 every two days. In four days the swelling was almost completely gone. Best food sources are fresh, raw fruits and vegetables, especially bananas, walnuts, filberts, peanuts, soybeans, sunflower seeds, fish, white chicken and lean muscle meat.

Instant Relief for Women's Problems!

One woman reports that her menopausal symptoms included hot flashes and extreme dryness of the vagina. She says:

"Even though I'm pushing 60, I don't like to discuss my still-active sex-life in print. But I must say that after taking a hormone pill for years, to control menopausal symptoms, I quit 'cold turkey' after reading of its cancer-causing dangers.

"Ever since, I've had awful hot flashes and also extreme dryness of the vagina that made intercourse painful. After hearing how vitamin E and calcium may relieve hot flashes, I tried them and, believe me, they worked! Even more amazing, to my great joy, I am once more encouraging my husband in bed instead of claiming I was 'tired,' as I'd been doing for months.

"I'd been too embarrassed to ask my doctor about this dryness—I haven't gone to him often and don't know him very well, and I find he tends to laugh off my aches and pains. But I'm really grateful to these miracle medicine foods for restoring my enjoyment of sex!"

Mrs. R.S. writes: "Two weeks before my period was due, I was the witch of all witches! My husband hated to even come home from work, and my poor kids—how they suffered! Oh yes, and I hated myself, too. I screamed at the kids for the littlest things and bit everyone's head off! I would get so depressed—suicidal. Then I tried brewer's yeast and vitamin B plus iron pills and believe me, what a change. My husband sure noticed the change, and I felt so much better towards life. To test this, I went for a month without them, and believe me, never again!"

A Miracle Medicine Food That Relieves Pain Immediately!

Pressing and rubbing certain nerves can be miracle medicine food for your body, often bringing dramatic relief from menstrual problems. It can stop practically all your aches and pains, in a matter of seconds, says one expert, induce anesthesia and allow a healing process to begin. In this manner, you can control painful menstruation like magic, without pills, relieve pain in the back and thighs. Many women hardly know when their period starts!

- A young girl had not menstruated in almost a year. She was given this miracle medicine food (nerve massage)—and in 5 minutes her period started, and she's had regular, normal, painless periods ever since!
- An older woman hadn't menstruated in over a year. She was given this miracle medicine food (nerve massage), and the next morning her period started and continued normally!
- One woman suffered a kidney ailment, and had an ovary so diseased she could hardly move. This miracle medicine food completely relieved her symptoms. She was also relieved of rectal pain which no longer bothered her!
- One woman who complained of painful spasms of the vagina (vaginismus) that made sex impossible, was told to try this miracle medicine food—nerve massage (massaging the hands and feet). She claimed the painful spasms and soreness were immediately relieved, and says it saved her marriage!

Massage for the ovaries below the outer ankle of each foot, or outer wrist of each hand. The uterus and vaginal canal are soothed by massaging below the inner ankle of each foot, or inner wrist of each hand. Nerve ends that lead to the kidneys are located in the middle of each palm and the middle of the underside of each foot. And those that lead to the rectum are located along the boney ridge of your palms and heels. These areas are rubbed until tenderness disappears.

Breast Tumor Disappeared!

One woman with two large breast tumors was about to have surgery. In the meantime, her doctor gave her this miracle medicine food—nerve massage—for immediate relief of pain. Specifically, she was instructed to press her tongue and wind rubber bands around her fingers. Pain was completely relieved. The nodes became so small, the doctor decided not to operate, and finally they disappeared!

(The reader is cautioned to seek qualified medical help immediately in any matters pertaining to the breasts. These items are presented solely as an aid to informed discussion. No cancer cure is claimed, and use of these remedies for self-medication is not permitted, without a doctor's consent.)

Uterine Fibroid Disappeared!

This same miracle medicine food (nerve massage) made a uterine fibroid disappear, and reduced painful glands in the neck, armpit, and groin, says this doctor. "While no claims are made to the effect that cancer can be cured by zone therapy (nerve massage), yet there are many cases in which pain has been completely relieved, and the patients freed from further use of opiates, and in a few cases the growths have also entirely disappeared," says this doctor.

Breast Cysts Relieved!

Robert London, M.D., director of obstetrical and gynecological research at Mount Sinai Hospital in Baltimore, Maryland, says that vitamin E can relieve fibrocystitis of the breasts (*Ob. Gyn. News*, December, 1976). Out of 12 menstruating women with fibrocystic breast disease, 10 improved in two months on 600 I.U of vitamin E daily. It seems to stimulate increased adrenal hormone secretion. No cure is claimed, but he says that it certainly seems to relieve lumps, sores and tenderness of the breasts, and no harmful side effects have been found.

Breast Lumps Disappeared!

Mrs. N.R. reports on another miracle medicine food: "Four months ago, I was diagnosed as having chronic cystic mastitis (breast cysts). At the time I went to see the doctor, I had controlled the cysts with dolomite. I did not tell him about it, but he said that the cysts were responding well to my hormones: that is to say, the cysts decreased in size and almost disappeared after each menstruation, only to reappear again after ovulation. (These were harmless.)

"Quite a few times I forgot to reorder more dolomite and had to suffer excessive pain, tenderness, and swelling in both breasts. But as soon as I would resume taking dolomite again, the pain and swelling would go away immediately.

"Without dolomite, I don't know what I'd do." Remember, dolomite contains calcium and magnesium. Experts have stated that calcium deficiency can produce swelling in the breasts and pain. Magnesium works with B-complex vitamins to soothe the nerves.

Double Breast Tumors Vanished
With Miracle Medicine Foods!

In his book, *Health Secrets from Europe* (Parker Publishing Co., Inc., 1970), Paavo Airola reports the case of Mrs. Elsa E., who was stricken with tumors in both breasts 17 years ago, at age 40. An examination at the Karolinska Institute in Stockholm showed that the lymphatic glands were also effected. Doctors insisted on an immediate operation the following week.

"I had no desire to be cut," says Mrs. E. Taking no chances, she decided to try another suggested method, while waiting for the operation. Her brother had informed her of the Waerland system, so during that week she went to see another doctor to ask him about it. On his advice, Mrs. E. started a treatment which consisted of short fasts and a raw juice diet. Then she was called to the Karolinska Institute for a final examination before the operation. After extensive examination, doctors, to their great surprise, could only declare that the tumors in both breasts had totally disappeared. There was no reason to operate![1]

---

[1] Apparently the doctors who wanted to operate in a week had themselves delayed the operation, for reasons not mentioned. Whatever the reason, Mrs. E. remained on the Waerland system, fasting on water and juices, for five weeks before being called for surgery.

Dr. Airola says that Mrs. E.'s case is well documented, with extensive examinations by renowned doctors. She visited the same hospital three to five times each year for the next five years for examination, with no evidence of any tumors. Sixteen years after her tumors were diagnosed, she was still, at age 56, in perfect health, free of disease. She faithfully continues the diet which saved her.

Dr. Airola summarizes the Waerland diet system as follows. On awakening in the morning, one-and-a-half cups of the Waerland drink, "Excelsior," a very alkaline drink composed of vegetable broth plus flaxseed and bran (a good laxative), is drunk seeds and all without chewing. This is followed by a head massage, a cold shower or rubdown with a sponge and drying with a rough towel, a drybrush massage all over, morning exercises of any type, a breakfast of homemade soured milk, yogurt or buttermilk in combination with fresh juicy fruits (apples, pears, grapefruit, oranges, bananas, grapes or fresh berries). No between-meal snacks are recommended, with the exception of fresh fruit or herb teas (any kind available at health stores) with honey as sweetener. For lunch, a bowl of Five-Grain Kruska, a cereal consisting of whole wheat, whole rye, whole oats, whole barley, whole millet, wheat bran, one tablespoon each, and two tablespoons unsulphured raisins. For dinner, a large bowl of fresh vegetable salad (green and leafy), a large portion of unpeeled potatoes (baked or broiled) and raw grated carrots, red beets and onions. Sour milk or yogurt are permitted, but no drinks of any kind. Cooked fruits can be used for dessert. Forbidden items include salt, vinegar, any sharp spices or condiments, coffee, tea, tobacco, alcohol, white sugar in any form (sweets), white bread, meat, fish, and eggs. During the first few days, enemas are recommended to relieve constipation. They should then be discontinued. This is the maintenance diet followed after water and raw juice therapy.

Poor Man's Penicillin Relieves Vaginal Infection!

One woman writes: "I am only 23 years old but for five years I suffered from an agonizing vaginal yeast infection. I saw a total of four doctors, the last one being a specialist. They gave me every remedy from purple dye to strong antibiotics, and at the same time, believe it or not, the good doctors told me antibiotics can cause yeast infection by killing off the good bacteria as well as the bad.... After reading that garlic acts like an antibiotic, I began to take fresh garlic cut up, and later on, manufactured garlic pills. I have found that, like an antibiotic, when I discontinue the garlic, the infection starts again. But there are two distinct advantages of taking the garlic (combined with vinegar douches) over the doctor-prescribed antibiotics. It is much cheaper and there are no side effects."

Monilia (Candida) Infection Cured With Miracle Medicine Foods!

Mrs. B.A. reports: "my problem was monilia (Candida) infection. I suffered with this for seven-and-one-half years, and five gynecologists could not cure it for me. Finally, the sixth doctor gave medication to both me and my husband. The following month I came down with a terrible viral infection and was given an antibiotic. Immediately, my monilia infection came back. Then I began taking frequent doses of acidophilus culture in pill form (available at health food stores), plus I began using plain yogurt instead of sour cream, and I cured my monilia."

Vaginitis-Cystitis Relieved!

Mrs. J.N. writes: "I would like to pass on... something that has brought relief from a 13-year problem with vaginitis-cystitis. I became prone to vaginal infections of various sorts in my late twenties. From that point on, although I was given a variety of prescriptions and pills and had examinations by both gynecologists and urologists, nothing helped. As I grew older and near menopausal time, the condition worsened.

> "Ultimately the infection from the vagina would lodge in the bladder, causing me much discomfort from frequency of urination. I was sent back and forth from the gyne-

cologist to the urologist, each telling me it was the opposite problem. Somewhere or other I had read about acidophilus yogurt and acidophilus tablets. I tried taking the tablets alone (eating commercial yogurt). That did not help. Then I read about inserting freshly made acidophilus yogurt directly into the vagina by means of a plastic applicator one can obtain in a drug store. . . .

Almost immedately my bladder symptoms abated and much of the vaginal irritation I had experienced for so long disappeared. It has been three months since I began this treatment and I have been delighted to find that I can travel, work and engage in activities without the constant desire to urinate, caused by vaginal infection. I have not been back to a doctor in this time. One last word: commercial yogurt will not work in this treatment. It must be freshly made acidophilus yogurt. . . . I purchased some acidophilus culture (making sure it was freshly dated) and made a batch. I inserted some at bedtime and also made sure I ate some of the yogurt daily."

Vaginal Yeast Problem Resolved!

Ms. W.R. reports: "About one year ago I got a vaginal yeast infection which caused me some discomfort. I got prescriptions for vaginal suppositories which I used for a total of five months—one prescription for 90 days straight, the other for 60 days. However, within a few weeks after discontinuing the medication, the infection would recur. Then I read an article about B vitamins . . . and decided to try them. I bought some B complex tablets and within two days the itching and inflammation was gone and has not recurred at all for the past three months."

Leukoplakia Cured!

Mrs. F.A. reports: "About five years ago, my mother, who was 80, developed leukoplakia inside and outside of her vaginal area. Her family doctor treated her with hormones, salve, etc. After a few weeks she became worse. I then took her to a specialist who treated her to no avail. Finally they informed me there was nothing else they could do.

"The specialist told me her system had dried out resulting from a complete hysterectomy which was performed 35 years prior to this ailment. (At that time the doctor did not prescribe hormones.) After eight or nine months, mother was in so much misery with her raw, burning area she could not sit, stand or walk in comfort.

"By the grace of God, I began thinking about vitamin E. I went to a health food store and got a bottle of vitamin E and gave her 200 units a day. After a few days she felt better. I was happy that she had relief, but was afraid to hope for recovery. In about a month's time her misery was completely gone. Mother is now 85 and doing very well."

Miracle Medicine Foods That Help Fight Anemia!

Anemia can be rapidly relieved by massaging the nerves that lead to the spleen (underside of the left foot, midway at the outer edge), says one expert. This happens with astonishing speed! As the liver and spleen are stimulated to produce new red blood cells, paleness, shortness of breath, palpitations of the heart and lack of energy are replaced with a rosy complexion, energy and a normal heartbeat. There are many types of anemia (some dangerous), which only a doctor can diagnose, these being the most common symptoms.

One woman claims that garlic cured her anemia! She says that eating this vegetable completely relieved her symptoms of weak digestion, numbness, tingling, fatigue, shortness of breath after slight exertion, pallor, lack of appetite, diarrhea, weight loss and fever.

With no complications, these are usually relieved with liver and vitamin B-12. But this woman says that garlic did it. She just couldn't seem to get enough of it and was never sick again after that "garlic binge." Let us now examine the unique factors present in garlic that may make it a miracle medicine food for many female complaints.

A Nearly All-Purpose Remedy!

Hot flashes? Try garlic. Feeling blue? Try a little garlic in your salad. Mild depression, irritability, anxiety, nausea, headache, tiredness or agitation, abdominal bloating, swelling of the extremities, dizziness, blurred vision, swelling and tenderness of the breasts, cramps, anemia, thyroid problems —all have been relieved by garlic, or substances that garlic contains. A proven emmenagogic, it stimulates the menstrual flow. It is an age-old remedy.

> **Today we know that garlic's ability to increase the body's absorption of vitamin B-1 may be of extreme value in relieving morning sickness, premenstrual tension, and more. Leading doctors have found that garlic brings relief from hot flashes, irritability, insomnia, palpitations, chills, itching, obesity, leucorrhea, arthritis and many other ailments.**

Garlic, of course, comes in powder, pill, or capsule form, available at most health food stores and herbal pharmacies. A tea is made simply by stirring a teaspoon of the powder in a cup of hot water, adding honey to taste. Or a small amount diced in a teaspoon of honey may be swallowed with water, before meals.

Reported Cases:
- **Mrs. L.D. writes: "I've always had menstrual cramps constantly the first two days of my period. But ever since taking garlic (about three months) I have hardly any. It's hard to believe, but it is the only thing I'm taking that I didn't take before that time. Now on each day of menstruation I take four or five garlic pills. I take two or three every day and, as said before, four or five on those difficult days.**
- **Harriet D., a 35-year-old housewife, suffered extreme weakness during her period, so extreme she could hard-**

ly do anything except lie still and not talk. She felt very shaky on her feet, with nervousness and trembling. She suffered cold sweats, extreme thirst, a feeling of faintness, and sometimes violent nausea and diarrhea. A friend suggested that she build up her resistance with garlic in her diet. To her surprise, each month she felt better and stronger. The trembling and nervousness disappeared, and she no longer dreads that time.

- Luanna B. said her pain was greatest on the right side, like a dragging and pressing downwards, starting in the back and spreading to the front, with bearing down pains that felt as if everything would fall out of her pelvis. She claimed this miracle rejuvenation plant gave her fast relief, as follows.

Inflammation Of The Uterus

The cramps a woman feels are usually muscular cramps from the emptying uterus during menstruation. The uterus can become inflamed. Another item of interest comes from Maurice Mességué, in his book *Of Men and Plants*. Here he gives a remedy for metritis (inflammation of the uterus). To use it, follow the directions in Chapter 2, page 37.

Garlic (one crushed head)
Single-seed hawthorn (crushed blossoms—one handful)
Greater celandine (leaves and stems, semi-fresh if possible—one handful)
Round-leaved mallow (flowers—one handful)
Blackberry brambles (leaves—one handful)
Sage (flowers and leaves—one handful)

This mixture is not to be eaten, and is for application only in the form of vaginal douches, or foot- and hand-baths.[2]

---

[2] Reprinted with permission of MacMillan Publishing Co., Inc. from *Of Men and Plants* by Maurice Mességué. Copyright © 1972 by Weidenfeld & Nicolson Ltd. Copyright © 1973 by Macmillan Publishing Co., Inc

Garlic and Morning Sickness

Remember that thiamin-boosting factor in garlic? Well, it has been found that the almost constant nausea and vomiting suffered by expectant mothers is completely relieved in many cases by thiamin (vitamin B-1). The *American Journal of Obstetrics and Gynecology* for August 1942 tells of a study in which complete relief was obtained by vitamin B-1 and B-6 injections. The dosage of B-1 was 25 to 100 mg. and the B-6 was usually 50 mg. The number of injections (and intervals between them) varied with individuals. Of 44 patients treated with thiamin, 39 experienced relief!

Complete relief of this condition was noted in an English study of constant vomiting among pregnant women. Each patient was given an intramuscular injection of 100 mg. of thiamin hydrochloride every other day.[3]

Remember that garlic increases the absorption of vitamin B-1 from food or other sources tenfold, *like liquid injections*. In the English study, fifty percent improvement was noted after the first injection. Within a week all patients gained weight on a general diet, without any recurrence of vomiting. If morning sickness is your problem, should you try garlic? That is for you and your doctor to decide. Garlic is a natural food that has been eaten by pregnant women even hours before delivery.

Red Raspberry Tea Relieved Labor Pains and Miscarriage Completely!

Violet Russell, M.D., wrote in *Lancet*, the British medical journal: "Somewhat shamefacedly, I have encouraged expectant mothers to drink this infusion. In a good many cases labor has been easy and free of muscular spasms." In one reported case, a woman had four miscarriages and despaired of ever having a child. Several doctors told her she could

---

[3] N. M. Marble, *Journal of the American Medical Association*, July 22, 1944.

never be a mother. A friend suggested this tea, which she drank every morning during pregnancy. She gave birth to a healthy baby, and in 18 months had another. In both cases labor was practically painless—so painless, in fact, that another woman who drank red raspberry tea was reading a paper only minutes before her baby was born!

Miracle Medicine Food Relieves Leg Cramps During Pregnancy!

Mrs. C.N. reports: "I used to have intense cramping in my legs every night for several years. They'd last ten to fifteen minutes, relieved somewhat by rubbing the calf of the leg and then gradually putting pressure on it by walking. Practically all the next day, I'd limp around with a tightness in the leg. But since I began taking 200 I.U. of vitamin E daily, I've been free of those 'nocturnal leg cramps' for over 13 years!

"I also found it extremely beneficial when I was pregnant and working full time. Being on my feet all day with the extra weight of the uterus cutting down circulation to my legs, I increased the dosage to 400 I.U. daily and experienced no cramps or 'painful legs.' I was even able to walk about a mile, most of it uphill, just a couple of hours before going into labor."

Rutin and Hemorrhoids!

Mrs. A.I. reports: "During all three of my pregnancies, I was in such pain with hemorrhoids that I nearly screamed with pain from something so simple as walking. Sitting or lying down became impossible. Then I sent my husband to the nearest natural foods health center for a bottle of rutin tablets. I began taking them immediately (I used three 50 mg. tablets a day). During an extremely restless night I finally must have fallen asleep.

"When I woke up in the morning the swelling had gone down considerably and by evening, I was able to sit down without wincing. In two day's time the swelling and pain were completely gone!

"Since that time I have been taking three tablets a day and haven't had a twinge of pain. It's been nearly a year and I can't believe it. I firmly believe this bioflavanoid compound really is a 'miracle' drug for me."

What Do We Mean By "Anemia?"

Anemia is common in women because of blood loss during menstruation, especially if the flow is heavy. It is also common in adolescent girls with bad diets, whose iron requirements are high because of muscle development. Anemia means that the body does not produce enough hemoglobin—the red oxygen-carrying substance in the blood. The chief complaints are weakness, dizziness, shortness of breath on exertion, palpitations, fatigue, and often brittle fingernails. Since too little oxygen gets to the brain, they cannot think clearly or quickly, and forget easily.

Hemoglobin—the blood substance which carries oxygen—cannot be produced without iron. Even a mild deficiency can result in headaches, fatigue, and shortness of breath. When persons with anemia eat beets, the red color is said to appear in the urine, which may be a good test for iron shortage!

Anemia can result from inadequate protein, iodine, cobalt, copper, vitamin C, or any of the B vitamins—all of which garlic and garlic foods contain.

Unique Factors Present In Garlic!

You may say that there aren't enough of any of these in garlic to affect most forms of anemia. However, there are these unique factors which may make garlic or foods that go well with garlic useful in such cases:

1. It isn't enough to eat iron-rich foods, or take iron supplements. It doesn't work unless there are enough B complex vitamins for the iron to be utilized. Garlic increases the absorption of B vitamins, especially vitamin B-1.
2. Copper, too, which garlic contains, is needed for iron assimilation. Also important, copper is needed for absorption and use of vitamin C from other foods.
3. Vitamin C vastly increases the assimilation of iron from food.

It is interesting to note that a deficiency in copper results in the same symptoms which occur when iron is deficient in supply, such as anemia, pale complexion, and a general weakened condition. Copper works with iron to produce hemoglobin—the red oxygen-carrying substance in the blood. You can be anemic because of lack of iron. But even if you start to take plenty of iron, you may still be anemic if there is not enough copper in your diet. In some cases, copper alone when added to the diet has relieved symptoms of iron deficiency. Garlic contains traces of copper—a trace mineral needed only in minutes quantities by the human body. Yet microscopic shortages can cause problems.

Kelp For Women's Anemia!

In a study of 400 obstetrical patients, it was found that the majority of these women were suffering from well-established secondary anemia. They were given kelp tablets (available at all health food stores) fortified with cobalt, manganese and folic acid. Within six to eight weeks on three tablets per day, the hemoglobin levels of their blood rose 85 percent. Furthermore, in patients who stopped taking the kelp, there was a rapid drop in hemoglobin levels, which rose again when the tablets were taken. In all patients studied there was a spectacular drop in the incidence of colds, and those who did catch colds had only light symptoms. In patients who came with a history of miscarriages, use of this supplement resulted in normal pregnancies in most cases.[4]

Miracle Medicine Foods
For Overweight & Goitres!

Studies have shown that women are more prone to overweight than men—especially at the menopausal stage. It is also during menopause that thyroid dysfunction is most evident. Symptoms of thyroid dysfunction—caused by lack of iodine—include sluggishness, overweight, or a goitre (which is a swelling of the thyroid gland at the base of the neck). Earlier in life, a thyroid deficiency may show up in the form of blinding, pressure headaches—starting around the age of 14—at the onset of each menstrual period. If allowed to progress, infertility may result, along with permanent ovary damage. It has been pointed out that many of these problems can be avoided with five cents' worth of iodine.

Ordinarily, you would think that the simplest solution would be to use iodized salt—but not if overweight is your problem. Many nutritionists feel that it is a mistake to add salt to food. The natural mineral salts in many foods (such as home-grown tomatoes) make them tasty enough. But more importantly, too much salt in the diet draws potassium out of the cells. Sodium (salt) enters, drawing in water, which is retained: Cells become waterlogged and the person appears overweight.

That's where garlic and kelp, in powder form, come in. Of all vegetables, these are the richest sources of iodine for the thyroid. They are also rich in potassium, which pulls out salt and releases excess fluid. They are delicious spices and are frequently used as salt substitutes by those on salt-restricted diets. They may be sprinkled on food, exactly like salt.

---

[4]G.L. Seifert and H.C. Woods, "The Use of Macrocystic Pyrifera as a Source of Trace Elements in Human Nutrition," a paper read at Second International Seawood Symposium, Trondheim, Norway, July 1955.

Thyroid Trouble Relieved!

Martha G. felt sluggish and overweight, due to a faulty thyroid gland. Her mind felt hazy, and she was forever dropping things. She gained weight easily and was always dieting, but could not seem to reduce, her hands felt clammy, her knees were weak, and at night her feet were cold. She felt "heat waves" every hour of the day. At times she had blinding headaches. The addition of garlic, kelp and plenty of seafood products to her diet relieved all her symptoms and made excess pounds melt away.

Fennel Tea For Overweight!

Fennel tea can help you shed unwanted pounds. In 1657, William Coles wrote, "Both the seeds, leaves, and roots of our garden fennel are much used in drinks and broths for those that are grown fat, to abate their unwieldiness and cause them to grow more gaunt and lank."

Reported Cases:
- One lady reported that she slimmed down from 210 to 140 lbs. with fennel tea: "I always drank four cups of the tea each day, one before breakfast, one on my 'coffee break,' one before dinner, and one just before going to bed. I did not follow a strict diet but just cut down a little on starches, sugars, and fats. Besides losing weight, I received an unexpected health benefit... after only 2½ months of drinking the tea I noticed that an old eye discomfort (bright light pained my eyes) had disappeared."[5]
- Another woman says: "I had a very stubborn weight problem, and tried dieting many times. I'd lose a few pounds at first, then for two or three weeks at a stretch I'd not lose another ounce even though I still followed my diet religiously. It was always at this point that my

---

[5] Richard Lucas, *The Magic of Herbs in Daily Living*, Parker Publishing Company, Inc., 1972.

poor will power would just give out and I'd start eating everything again. Then one day a friend suggested I try powdered fennel seed. I don't know if it would help others with a stubborn weight problem but it certainly did marvels for me. When I went back on my diet and took the capsules of powdered fennel seed my weight dropped steadily—no more episodes of trying to struggle through periods where the pounds just wouldn't come off. I have been down to my normal weight for some time now and I find that I can be fairly liberal in my eating habits without gaining, so long as I keep taking my capsules of powdered fennel seed. I have also noticed that fennel has done wonders for my digestion."[6]

Other Miracle Medicine Foods For Quick Weight Loss!

Other weight reducing foods include cleavers. A medical herbalist reported the case of an overweight woman who drank this herbal tea daily. The first month nothing happened, but in the fifth week she began to lose weight. In six months she lost a total of 32 pounds and has not put back an ounce.[7]

Apple cider vinegar contains powerful enzymes that help dissolve clumps of fat, and wash them right out of the system—so powerful, in fact, that meat soaked in apple cider vinegar is tenderized. When you drink it, even in such small quantities as two tablespoons in fruit or vegetable juice, moments later it is breaking up accumulated fat in cell tissues, says one expert.[8]

Cleopatra won a bet when she dissolved pearls in vinegar, and reportedly it can dissolve solid fat in the body! (Sauerkraut is another food which can do this.)

---

[6] Lucas, *Op. cit.*
[7] Lucas, *Ibid.*
[8] Carlson Wade, *The New Enzyme-Catalyst Diet,* Parker Publishing Company, Inc., 1976.

Breast Surgery Avoided!

Once again, we stress the power of positive thought as miracle medicine food for your body. In her book, *The Miracle of Metaphysical Healing* (Parker Publishing Co. Inc., 1975), Evelyn Monohan tells of Jean L. who had just learned that she would have to undergo surgery for the removal of a nonmalignant tumor. Her husband asked if Miss Monohan would help, and was told of the method of positive thought she was to use three times a day. Miss Monohan says this method is 100 percent effective. It involves clearly visualizing the disease you wish cured, in a quiet place, relaxed, with eyes closed, and visualizing it fading away, with positive affirmations that you will be cured, completely blotting out any negative thoughts, for 15 minutes a day. Three days later, Jean's husband called to report the exciting news: Jean's tumor dissolved and she would not need surgery!

13

Miracle Medicine Foods For Men's Problems!

Prostate trouble! The mere thought of it strikes terror in the heart of every man, starting at about the age of fifty—often even younger. The visions it conjures up, such as sterility, impotence, pain, catheterization, the wearing of a Foley bag, surgery and even death, are unfortunately justifiable.

First Signs Of Prostate Enlargement

David J. first began to suspect that he had prostate trouble when he had difficulty urinating. Frequent urges, a feeling of incompleteness each time, and just a dribble or diminution of stream when he finally went—these were signs that something was wrong. Occasionally, he'd experience a burst of pain just before urinating. And there were frequent pains in the lower part of his back, burning on urination, and urinary infections. A medical diagnosis confirmed it: prostatic hypertrophy (an enlarged prostate).

Feeble Attempts At Relief

Prostate massages, administered by a doctor, did not seem to help much, and were very painful. He was given a number of drugs to help clear up the infections, and thence the burning. The bursting sensation prior to urination was quite painful. He soon discovered that if he went on a long trip, he had to schedule his stops. If he drove a car, he found the sitting position (tilted slightly back) relieved it to the point that he felt normal and wasn't really aware that he had to urinate until he stood up. At night, there were endless trips to the bathroom. Excitement, a violent argument, or emotional situations of any kind would give him a tremendous urge to urinate. And when he got there, the tension alone would prevent him from doing so.

The Alternatives

The symptoms came and went. David was terrified of real trouble—complete blockage or inability to urinate. He'd heard cases of people dying from prostate surgery. He knew there were three kinds of operations—and he knew of people who had them: intra-urinary, ennucleation and radical.

Briefly, the urethra—carrying urine from the bladder—comes down and, in effect, through the prostate. And if the prostate enlarges, it cuts off the flow of urine. Prolonged enlargement and irritation can lead to infection (due to toxic material in the prostate) and the backup of urine to the kidneys, hence real trouble.

In intra-urinary surgery, the surgeon inserts a catheter into the penis, until it reaches and probes inside the prostate. With the tip of a special instrument, the doctor cauterizes the inner lining of the prostate, bit by bit, hopefully until there's just a shell left. Sometimes however, they don't get all of it, and that calls for repeated attempts. A friend of David's who'd undergone this complained of much pain afterward for several weeks, and also an infection of the occipital gland at the base of the spine.

In ennucleation, the surgeon enters either topside (suprapubic) or through the rectum, and carves out the lining of the prostate, leaving a shell through which urine flows. (Eventually, a crystalline tube—a continuation of the uretha—forms again through this gland after several months. In the meantime, urine actually flows through the gland, which expands or collapses accordingly.)

Either way, he'd heard, the man is always rendered sterile and often impotent (it is the prostate gland which manufactures and holds like a resorvoir the seminal fluid, into which sperm from the testicles are ejaculated in coitus).

The ultimate terror was radical surgery—when cancer is suspected—in which the prostate is completely removed, and the uretha connected directly to the bladder.[1] In terms of prostate trouble, you know you've had it—David knew—and are due for surgery, when you've been hospitalized once or twice, and have had to wear a Foley bag for a while. The mere thought of catheterization sent shudders through him.

A Little-Known Method Of Relief

Fortunately, he had not reached this point yet. It was then that I managed to convince him to try the garlic diet, outlined below. Many ailments, I reasoned, have a way of subsiding as excess pounds melt away. David J. was about forty pounds overweight. Even if you're not overweight, a program of natural foods and natural living has a way of detoxifying the system, relieving ailments that range from intestinal trouble to high blood pressure, kidney trouble and even arthritis.[2]

My own ulcer healed, after a good diet—as did my hemorrhoids which always seemed to flare up whenever I gained weight. I even had symptoms of prostatitis and urinary infections (all diagnosed by a doctor) which cleared up on this diet. David J. took my advice, and soon began experiencing the relief he had hoped for. Gone were the urinary infections, the pain and burning, the frequent trips to the bathroom and the feeling of incompleteness. I am intimately familiar with this cure, of course, since I used it myself.

---

[1] There is now yet another method for treating an enlarged prostate. Doctors have discovered that one way of shrinking the prostate is by hormone therapy—the absence of male hormones or presence of female hormones seems to help, except in advanced cases. The danger of this method, of course, is that the man will develop enlarge breasts and other female characteristics.

[2] Max Warmbrand, *How Thousands of My Arthritis Patients Regained Their Health*, (West Nyack, N.Y.: Parker Publishing Company, Inc.), 1970.

The Garlic Diet

The garlic diet is like no other diet you have ever seen before. Although I never count calories, I would assume it's around 750 or 800 calories a day—but it doesn't *seem* like a diet at all!

The major feature of the garlic diet is that it is extremely well-rounded, giving you large, generous portions of food at lunch and supper, every day, from each of the five major categories of food, so that you never miss out on anything. Meats, fish, poultry, fruits and vegetables—all are included as well as delicious diet snacks between meals!

The basic diet I followed even contained fruit, cake, or candy every day. And lots and lots of garlic! Nowadays, as I mentioned before, it is possible to achieve the same results without the slightest trace of garlic breath simply by taking a garlic capsule before each meal, instead. So if eating garlic is not to your taste, simply omit it from your menu.

BREAKFAST:
>An orange or grapefruit (grapefruit may be sweetened with sugar substitute).
>A slice of toast or bread rubbed with garlic.
>Tea or coffee, with milk.

LUNCH:
>A hamburger, *or*
>A piece of chicken (legs, breasts, wings) *or*
>Tuna fish in a container, mixed with a dash of mayonnaise or diet mayonnaise—if desired—diced garlic or onion and bits of celery.
>A small container of salad, with lots of garlic.
>A small piece of fruit—a plum, an apple, half orange, a pear, or half a cantaloupe. (Pick one).
>One piece of candy, *or*
>Several low calorie candies, *or*
>Small slice of plain cake of any kind, *or*
>One or two small cookies or crackers.
>Tea or coffee, with milk, or a low-calorie soda.

SUPPER:
>A leafy green salad, mixed with diced garlic or onion.
>One or two vegetables (one portion each).
>One portion of steak or chicken or fish.
>A small piece of fruit—see lunch—*or*
>One piece of candy, *or*
>Several low calorie candies, *or*
>Small slice of plain cake of any kind, *or*
>One or two small cookies, or crackers, *or*
>Jello (regular *or* low-calorie, any flavor).
>Tea or coffee, with milk, or a low-calorie soda.

Try to vary your meals as much as possible. Have an additional portion of any meat, fish, poultry, salad or vegetable—at any meal—if desired. Concentrate on green, leafy vegetables, cabbage, green beans, spinach, kale, brussels sprouts, broccoli spears—garlic foods (foods that go well with garlic). You may even use margarine or diet margarine on them for flavor if your diet permits. Steer clear of baked beans, lima beans, peas, corn, potatoes of any kind, and—if the fruit category—bananas, as these are high in starches and calories. However, once or twice a week it is permissible to sneak these things in at lunch or supper—no harm is done. For salads, use lots of tomatoes, green peppers, lettuce, celery, and carrots. You may use vinegar or any non-fattening salad dressing or a dash of mayonnaise. One slice of bread is permitted at any meal, provide the cake is omitted.

Between lunch and supper, and after supper, typical snacks might include Jello, one or two handfuls of soybeans or sunflower seeds, fruit—in other words, one or two of the desserts you did not pick for lunch or supper. Don't overdo it. Have one short snack between meals and stop.

Additional Pointers

Use salt sparingly—or use a salt substitute or even garlic powder in place of salt. Of the fishes, the best fish to eat is codfish or halibut, because they are lower in calories. Filet of flounder won't hurt you (assuming fried foods agree with you). Pork and lamb are the only meats I avoided. They slowed down the weight loss. And I always took two multi-vitamin tablets in a yeast base daily to guard against stress.

Once a week or so, you can have a bit of rice (half a cup) or spaghetti or French fries (half a cup). Mushrooms may be eaten by the can or mixed with rice or vegetables—they are low in calories. Most normal condiments, such as ketchup, mustard or horseradish, are fine. Relish and pickles are a little high in salt, but fine in moderation. Sauerkraut is very low in calories and perfectly acceptable.

That's all there is, basically, to this excellent reducing diet. There were no low-calorie candies and salad dressings when I first tried this years ago, and low-calorie beverages were just coming out. Of course, you have to cut your fluid intake—you can't drink gallons and gallons of different things—but you *can* fill up, between meals, on diet soft drinks in moderation. Medical people say you're supposed to have six glasses of water a day, but few people can drink that much. You get water in your coffee or tea and in your foods as well.

Recently, a national newspaper told how a famous actor—we'll call him John L.—uses garlic in another way to lose weight fast. For breakfast he would have a glass of juice (orange or grapefruit), one piece of dry toast and a cup of black coffee; for lunch, a large salad of endive and lettuce smothered in oil and vinegar and loaded with garlic, or grated celery or carrots (raw), covered with garlic dressing. Dinner was a healthy portion of meat, sliced tomatoes doused with garlic dressing, an occasional baked potato and a glass of wine. A consulting dietician said the diet is medically safe, but suggested adding a slice of enriched bread. "I can lose a pound and a half a day," says this actor. That's about ten pounds a week! While making a movie, he had to lose 20 pounds and did in twelve days with this amazing diet.

Either way, it's been my experience that pounds seem to melt away faster than anything else in the world with this diet. Best of all, it seems to melt off pounds in all the right places: thighs, hips, buttocks, neck—all the hard-to-reach areas—seem to "slenderize." Even shoe size is reduced. Skin on face, throat, and arms appears taut, smooth, and young-looking. Wrinkles seem to fade away!

Can The Garlic Diet Heal A Prostate?

Frankly, I do not know if it was the garlic, the diet, or the lessening of pressure on internal organs that relieved it. All I know is that afterwards, the condition seemed completely healed, and never returned. There is good reason, however, to believe that the mineral and chemical content of garlic might have something to do with healing the prostate.

First, of course, there is sulfur content. Compounds of sulfur—which are responsible for garlic's strong smell—have the power to fight germs and infection. Pharmaceuticals (prescribed drugs) used to combat urinary infections, such as Furadantin, often contain sulfur.

This is important because, as described in Gray's *Anatomy:* "In consequence of the enlargement of the prostate a pouch is formed at the base of the bladder behind the projection, in which water collects and cannot entirely be expelled. It becomes decomposed and ammoniacal, and leads to crystitis" (the formation of crystals in the bladder, symptoms of which are pain and infection).

This, in turn, can affect the kidneys and lead to a buildup of urinary wastes in the bloodstream. Garlic detoxifies the system, neutralizes and cleanses poisons with a penetrative power that pervades the entire body.

How A Mineral In Garlic Relieved Prostate Trouble!

In a report entitled, "Zinc: A Key Urological Element," Dr. Irving M. Bush and his associates make a number of interesting points. One is that after checking a total of 210 healthy men of various ages, "seven percent of males have low semen and prostatic zinc levels. In addition, 30 percent of males may have borderline values." Thirty-seven percent! Quite a large figure.

Can zinc be used as a treatment or cure? Dr. Bush and his associates tried it on 194 patients suffering from various illnesses of the prostate, including 32 with cancer. Here are the results:

- **In chronic prostatitis, treatment with zinc for two to 16 weeks relieved the symptoms in 70 percent of the 40 patients treated. (Other treatments did not help at all.**
- **Fifteen patients with simple enlargement of the prostate all reported improvement. After two months of treatment, actual shrinkage of the prostate occurred in some!**

The garlic diet will give you zinc—in garlic and plenty of other natural foods—over a period of time that corresponds to lengths of treatment cited (two to three months), depending on how much weight you wish to lose. But even if you're not overweight, and wish to try it as a means of detoxifying the system, it seems perfectly safe. In that case you can add certain foods.

You'll get plenty of zinc in your diet. In addition to garlic and onion, zinc-rich foods include brewer's yeast, nuts, molasses, eggs, rice bran, rabbit, chicken, peas, beans, lentils, wheat germ, wheat bran, beef liver and gelatin. The meat and vegetables go especially well with garlic.

Experiments Show Genitals Grow Larger!

In a study written up in both the *Archives of Internal Medicine* (volume 407, 1963) and the *American Journal of Clinical Nutrition* (December 1966), Dr. A.A. Prasad and his associates found that 40 boys admitted to the research ward of the U.S. Naval Medical Research Unit in Cairo suffered both growth retardation and hypogonadism. The report was titled, "Zinc Levels and Blood Enzyme Activities in Egyptian Male Subjects with Retarded Growth and Sexual Development," and showed that these boys were not only short—they also lacked facial or pubic hair and had the genitals of children.

They also suffered a profound zinc deficiency. All were treated with does of zinc sulfate and put on good diets.

Almost immediately their genitals began to develop to normal size. The most amazing change was in growth rate. The shortest was 20 years old and only 39 inches tall. He grew five inches in a matter of months!

The level of zinc in their blood and hair rose to normal levels. All of which leads up to the two richest sources of zinc in common foods.

Miracle Medicine Foods For Prostate Disorders!

Sunflower seeds and pumpkin seeds are the richest sources of zinc available in common foods. Sunflower seeds seem to have a normalizing effect in disorders of the prostate gland. The reports indicate strongly that this is due to their unsaturated fatty acid content in combination with other factors. The main reason why pumpkin seeds are indicated for prostate health is their high zinc content. Dr. W. Devrient of Berlin, Germany, reports that he has been curing patients of prostatic trouble by having them eat pumpkin seeds regularly. They can be eaten like candy.

Prostate and Hernia Relieved!

Another word on this important mineral comes from Mrs. Emma G., of Silver Springs, Maryland:

> "My husband had been having trouble with swelling and discomfort of the prostate gland, giving him a great deal of misery. I started him on a program of zinc—and the results were beyond our expectations. Not only did he have immediate relief, but a byproduct of the treatment seems to be relief of excess acidity caused by an esophagus hernia he has been suffering for years! I don't understand what happened or why, but the results are amazing. We are both very grateful."

And Mr. V.W., of Auburn, Washington, states: "About three years ago, I was told through a physical that I had an enlarged prostate. I have taken vitamins and minerals for the last year. A nutritionist recommended that in addition to these supplements and diet that I take zinc, vitamin F and polly seeds. Lo and behold, a medical doctor checked me out and told me that I had no more prostate trouble!"

Prostate Completely Relieved!

Mr. N.R. reports: "When I heard that zinc helps the prostate problem I decided on taking a zinc tablet every day. I used to get up once or twice during the night, but since I am taking the zinc tablets, at the age of 72, I can sleep eight to nine hours without ever getting out of bed. That's great!"

Prostate Relieved, Surgery Avoided With Miracle Medicine Food!

Mr. N.J. reports: "Even though I have a vitamin-conscious M.D. who placed me on B complex vitamins daily, I began to suffer prostate trouble. So to the vitamins I was taking I added bee pollen which I'd been reading about. My urologist had been suggesting a prostate gland removal but after a pyelogram x-ray, he told me that I had improved. He said there was still some enlargement of the prostate but not enough to cause any distress. I believe that adding bee pollen to my other vitamins and changing to a more nutritious diet helped my prostate to start returning to normal. I still eat bee pollen. I am 70 years of age and walk at least three miles out in the air every day."

Miraculous Relief Of Prostate!

Mr. A.C. reports: "A few months ago, I heard how pollen helps prostate problems. I decided to take two tablets a day and after two weeks all symptoms disappeared. No urologists, no sitz baths, no discomfort at all after eleven years—a miracle."

Herpes Genitalis Relieved!

Mr. A.L. reports: "During the past eleven years I have been plagued with a presently incurable disease known as 'herpes-2' or 'herpes genitalis.' This seems to be a virus related to chicken pox. It is characterized by a cluster of blisters erupting on the skin of the penis, over a nerve path. These get painful, and within a week they break open and drain; then they form scabs and heal up. They may then recur the following week, or month, at random, but I was never free from them for periods exceeding four months (until the past year).

"Needless to say, besides being extremely painful it interferes greatly with a normal sex life. Science cannot detect this virus in its dormant stage, and has nothing in the way of a cure except antiseptics during the stage of open sores.

"Now, for all those who are, like I was, without hope, I have discovered a virtual *miracle:* a little more than a year ago I was introduced to zinc supplements, and I thought I would try it, along with my other vitamins and minerals (to improve my health and well-being, but with *no* thought to the herpes). I bought a bottle of 100 tablets (each tablet is 50 mg. of elemental zinc in 348 mg. of zinc gluconate), and began taking one per day. To my amazement, after trying everything and going to countless doctors for ten years, I did not have a single outbreak of herpes. I hardly dared to believe it, so, at the end of 100 days I stopped taking them (when I ran out) for about a week! *During this period the herpes recurred!*

"I promptly bought 250 more zinc tablets, and have been taking them ever since (about eight months now) and have not had *one* further attack of herpes! Complete relief!

"This is good enough for me. I believe that when the human system has enough zinc to work with it can somehow keep this virus dormant. (Science believe that almost everyone has this virus, although it remains dormant in most people.)

"I know that I shall never again be without zinc, and I hope many others will find the same relief I did."

Another Miracle Medicine Food For Genital Herpes!

Mr. E.N. reports: "About a year ago. I contracted *herpes genitalis,* and found no cure. Then I heard about taking vitamin B-12 for herpes. I bought some at my local health food store—and within ten days, after taking 300 mg. daily, practically all of the symptoms disappeared. Since then there have been two recurrences of the vague deep pain (one of several symptoms) but no blisters, no eruptions, no redness and tenderness. By any comparison I am cured."

Embarrassing Impotence Miraculously Cured!

Albert J., 65, was extremely depressed due to impotence, which he associated with old age and loss of his manhood. A visit to the doctor left him even more depressed. The doctor told him it was all part of the "old age syndrome" (he had never thought of himself as old), and told him to try to "think positive." There was nothing organically wrong, the doctor said; rather, it was a symptom of mental depression of some sort. "You mean I'm getting senile?" "Not exactly," the doctor said, but Albert wasn't at all convinced. He feared the loss of other faculties as well, and pictured himself as a withered old man. The doctor wasn't much help, it seemed. He even warned Albert about the dangers of taking artificial stimulants, because they could inflame the whole urinary tract. "But I feel like an old man," said Albert. "I don't want to be old before my time! I've just retired. I want to enjoy life!"

Then Albert read how garlic makes great lovers better, how the ancient Greeks and Romans used it as a restorer of masculine vigor. It increased the absorption of B vitamins tenfold, an amount heretofore impossible except by liquid injections. B vitamins were given at expensive

health spas and rejuvenation clinics, to combat aging symptoms; B vitamins are important for healthy nerves. Specifically, he read how garlic stimulates the central nerve of the penis and helps cause erection... and how it stimulates the hormone glands as well, for long-lasting sexual power!

He read how pumpkin seeds supply the male organs with zinc, affording dramatic relief from prostate trouble and impotence! Albert began including garlic and pumpkin seeds in his diet every chance he got, and took his garlic capsules regularly. Almost immediately, he could feel new-found strength surging through his body. His wife was astonished and quite excited. The impotence vanished, and never occurred again—and Albert sings the praises of garlic for his cure!

Amazing New Prostate Massage Brings Relief from Embarrassing Male Problems, Instantly!

In this case, we are talking about nerve massage, and *not* the type of massage doctors normally use, which can be very painful and embarrassing. You needn't get undressed to use it—or even touch the area involved—and you can do it yourself, any time, easily.

One expert claims 100 percent relief, in every case treated. It's safe and easy. To soothe a prostate, massage the cord above the heel and just below the inner ankle on each foot, or the inner wrist above the palm of each hand. The testicles may be relieved by massaging the outer wrist of each hand, or just below the outer ankle of each foot, until all pain and tenderness disappear.

This a perfectly harmless method of massaging the nerves that lead to the sex glands, causing anesthesia, blessed relief from pain, and often complete cures! The stimulation afforded by healing nerve massage can be miracle medicine food for your body!

Reported Cases:
- A man with an enlarged prostate gland, with burning and scalding urine and pus, went to a doctor and was given a series of painful prostate massages by way of the rectum—so painful he nearly passed out each time. The burning and scalding returned. But when he used this miracle medicine food (nerve massage), the burning disappeared and never returned!
- A 36-year-old man awoke one morning with excruciating pain in his left testicle. It was constant and refused to subside for three weeks. He couldn't stand, walk or sit properly, and feared cancer. His doctor felt no lumps and said it was just an inflamation (epididymitis). He was told to rest, with his testicle raised, with warm applications. This gave no relief. With the miracle medicine food, he massaged his left outer wrist (which was tender) and noticed his testicle stopped hurting, in seconds! He has had no further trouble!
- A man noticed a strange feeling in his testicle, like fluid moving around. His scrotum was swollen, and it was very annoying, with a heavy dragging feeling, worse if he walked, or exercised. His doctor said it was enlarged or varicose veins (varicocele), a mild case. The best treatment was to ignore it, he said. Or wear a support. It was caused by too much pressure during constipation. He was given a laxative. Nothing helped. He then tried these miracle medicine foods: nerve massage and bran for regularity, and felt immediate relief from the swelling and heavy dragging feeling.
- A 50-year-old man with a wife described as very passionate, was impotent and felt humiliated by his condition. He tried this miracle medicine food—nerve massage—and felt a sudden surge of power such as he had not felt in 20 years, and the embarassing condition never returned! He did this by massaging the penis nerve on the inner wrist of each hand and below the inner ankle of each foot, and the testicles and prostate as described above.
- One man suffering impotence due to premature ejaculation says his wife was becoming very dissatisfied. He

tried this miracle medicine food, to stimulate the central nerve of the penis and found it not only cured his impotence but turned ordinary love-making into hours of ecstasy! (All the male organs were massaged as described above.)

The reader is cautioned to seek immediate medical advice in all matters pertaining to the male sex glands. Failure to do so can result in serious conditions that only a doctor can diagnose and treat. Self medication is not permitted without a doctor's consent.

14

Miracle Medicine Foods For The Skin

In this chapter, you'll see how a man who was horribly scalded from head to foot by boiling water received immediate, instant, and complete relief—and escaped completely unharmed—with a miracle medicine food!

You'll see how a woman with thousands of ugly black warts all over her face, neck and chest made them vanish! How a diabetic's incurable skin condition was completely healed! How gangrene of the foot vanished and horrible leg ulcers healed!

You'll see how dozens of other common and uncommon skin ailments were quickly, easily, and completely healed with miracle medicine foods, many of which you have stored in your kitchen cabinets right now! Instant relief for skin problems!

Miraculous Healing With Honey!

Because of its hygroscopic or water-attracting properties, honey has been found to be a good healer of wounds and burns. Disease-producing germs cannot live without water, which reportedly makes honey an excellent germ-killer.

One man reports: "In the winter of 1933 I heated a boiler of about 35 gallons of water. When I opened the cover,

it flew with great force against the ceiling. The vapor and hot water poured forth over my unprotected head, over my hands and feet. Some minutes afterwards I had violent pains and I believe I would have gone mad if my wife and daughter had not helped immediately.

"They took large pieces of linen, daubed them thickly with honey and put them on my head, neck, hands and feet. Instantly the pain ceased. I slept well all night and did not lose a single hair on my head. When the physician came to see me he shook his head and said, 'How can such a thing be possible?' "

Other Reported Cases:
- An elderly woman was admitted to a hospital with gangrene of the foot, but after examining her the doctors decided she could not survive an amputation. It was decided to try honey. Her foot was literally tied in a bag of honey. To everyone's amazement, the foot soon healed, and she walked out of the hospital on her own power! She remains well!
- Another woman had a horrible case of chickenpox. She was covered from head to foot with spots. Remembering the healing power of honey, she smeared some over her entire body, covered herself with towelling, and went to bed. In three days, she felt perfectly well, the chickenpox was gone, and her skin was completely smooth and clear!
- One man had a large carbuncle on his back. It was operated on by a surgeon and left a deep ugly scar. Then he developed another. This he treated only with honey. Although enormous in size, the second carbuncle rapidly disappeared, leaving only a tiny dot!
- A lady reports that while brewing some coffee for guests, she accidentally spilled the entire pot of boiling water on her thigh. Without telling anyone, she managed to get to the kitchen, in agony. There, she covered the burned area with lots of honey, and wrapped a clean towel around her leg. In a few seconds, the pain was gone. She returned to the party in a clean skirt as

if nothing had happened. The pain had gone away so completely that she forgot about it and slept soundly that night. Next morning, removing the dressing, she found a huge blister—bigger than two hands—but repeated applications of honey soon healed it!

It is reported that ulcerated legs from varicose veins do not heal easily, particularly in the elderly, but that regular daily application of honey can soon reduce the infection and bring a complete healing! It is said that an amazingly effective remedy for erysipelas is to cover the area—and a little beyond—with lots of honey, dress with cotton, and allow to remain for 24 hours, repeating as necessary. In the jungles of South America, doctors smear honey over raw open wounds after surgery, with excellent results. Honey is truly a miracle medicine food!

Lipoma Tumors and Sebaceous Cyst Heal, Avoiding Surgery!

Mrs. H.N. reports: "For many years I have been subject to lipoma tumors and have had to undergo several operations ... as they were inhibiting the circulation in my joints (especially the knee). Three years ago I underwent surgery in my right chest for a lipoma which was growing between the lungs and against the heart. The surgeons told me ... that I had a crack on the diaphragm and that a growth of fat had developed through this crack and was growing in the chest cavity. (Recently I noticed a growth in my ankle.)

> "These are considered non-malignant but can cause an obstruction in the circulation. Since I have been taking lecithin and vitamin C, I have noticed quite an improvement. The growth near the ankle has gone, a bump between two of my ribs (sebaceous cyst) has almost gone. I attribute this to taking the lecithin and vitamin C.

"There is one other thing I would like to mention. For a number of years I have been bothered by a peculiar skin eruption which was seen on the inner arms near the elbow joint. I went to a dermatologist who said it was due to a deep-seated emotional disturbance. I strongly felt that that was not the cause of the eruption. Since taking a capsule containing vitamin A with vitamin D in the form of three fish oils, I have gotten rid of this eruption. . . . I had a vitamin deficiency all the time."

Dog's Breast Tumors Disappear!

Mrs. K.N. reports: "Our poodle had breast tumors that the vet said were probably malignant and should be removed. I had just read an article on garlic, so I started her on four perles a day. Three weeks later the tumors had disappeared. She now takes garlic daily." Two years later, Mrs. K.N. reported the dog to be still alive and healthy!

Diabetic Skin Ailment Cured With Miracle Medicine Food!

Ms. R.L. writes: "Several years ago I developed an allergy to a very common insulin which caused flesh to disappear at the site of injections, creating 'dents' or 'craters' ranging in size from very small dimples to very large areas the size and depth of the palm of my hand. They were all over my body and very unsightly. I was told by the specialist . . . that he had consulted with experts in diabetes and they agreed that these wasted areas would never return to their former condition. . . .

"For over a year I did nothing for this wasted condition, believing nothing was possible. One day, accidentally, I discovered the solution. Having very dry skin, I had rubbed peanut oil all over my body. All of a sudden I noticed that at the bottom of each 'dent' the skin was dry as a bone, while the rest of the skin area had not yet absorbed the oil. I put more oil in each dent and watched.

"Almost immediately the oil was absorbed. I continued applying oil daily, several times. In addition, I would massage and pound the normal area around each dent, and gradually they began to smooth out. I was very careful never to touch or apply pressure to the inside or bottom of any of the dents. Another accidental discovery followed. I gained approximately five pounds, kept it on for a couple of months, and then lost it. Each time I did this, I noticed that the bottom of each dent was filling up gradually with flesh. I deliberately continued this alteration of weight loss and gain. Now, I have only a couple of small reminders of the formerly severe condition. It took me approximately two years to do this. I feel, however, that if a person started it immediately after the condition developed, it would probably not take so long to cure. . . .

"The first dents to disappear were two large ones on my stomach. The next to go was an enormous one the size and depth of the palm of my hand which was located on my right leg. I told my doctor what I was doing; he did not believe me until he examined me and discovered that the incurable condition no longer existed. I do not know whether he passed along my discovery or not, but I felt that I should let other diabetics know that this is not hopeless and can be overcome. I think that about 200 diabetics out of 1000 are afflicted with this alergy. Peanut oil seems to work better than other oils, and much faster. Later, I read that the psychic, Edgar Cayce, recommended peanut oil for 'wastage of flesh' and that it would even smooth out scar tissue. I hope this information is of help. It works! It takes time, the faithful application of oil, massage, and weight gain and loss of a few pounds, but it works and returns the flesh to normal."

Disgusting Ulcers Vanish!

It has been stated that, "A poultice of (carrot) roots has been found to mitigate the pain of foul cancerous ulcers, and take away the intolerable stench. . . ." As a salve for ulcerated areas, an amount of the juice of carrot root is evaporated slowly on very low heat to a consistency of thick syrup. This liquid is then applied to ulcerated areas, or simply use thin slices of the root as an external poultice, as needed.

The common herb comfrey seems to possess extraordinary healing powers. This is all due to a substance it

contains called *allantoin*. It is used as a poultice or tea drink, and doctors have used its medicinal extract in cases of stubborn ulcers, burns, and open wounds, with dramatic and stunning results!

W. Turner's *Herball* (1568) states: "Of Comfrey ... the rootes are good if they be broken and drunken for them that spitte blood, and are bursten. The same layd to, are good to glewe together freshe wounds (it is used in bone setting). They are also good to be layed to inflammation..." Gerard's *Herball* (1597) states that comfrey is effective in healing up "ulcers of the lunges" and "ulcers of the kidneys, though they have been of long continuance." Parkinson's *Theatrum Botanicum* (1640) adds: "The roots of comfrey, taken fresh, beaten small, spread upon leather, and laid upon any place troubled with gout, does presently give ease of the paines; and applied in the same manner, give the ease to pained joints, and profiteth very much running and moist ulcers, gangrenes, mortifications, and the like."

Reported Cases:
- A doctor reports the case of a man, age 83, suffering from a number of serious ailments, including a loud heart murmur, a feeble pulse, advanced hardening of the arteries, shortness of breath and swelling of the legs. Suddenly a large fulminating ulcer appeared on his left foot. It spread rapidly—exposing the bones. His condition looked hopeless, he became delirious, and was taken home to die. There he was treated with four-hourly fomentations made with a decoction of comfrey root. The ulcer immediately began to fill up rapidly and was almost completely healed in a month, and all his other symptoms improved!
- Another doctor reports the case of a woman with a large, gangrenous ulcer full of pus covering the lower part of her leg. He was thinking of amputating her leg —the ulcer was about five inches wide, and had been there five years. Extract of comfrey (allantoin) was applied in dressings. A week later, islands of healing appeared. In 23 days, this huge ulcer was reduced to

the size of a pin head, and the patient was sound and well!

- Mrs. R.E. reports: "I was suffering with ulcers on both legs. These ulcers started out like blisters. If they go untreated until after they break and start oozing, they spread fast. I was doing a lot of praying to God for help. They wanted to put me in the hospital but I wouldn't go. The treatment the doctor wanted me to use made my legs feel like they were on fire. He said I'd have to have a skin graft also. I said no. Then I read about dried comfrey root, and bought some at a health food store. I made tea by pouring scalding water on it in a quart fruit jar; I drank it and also washed the ulcer with it. When the root had softened enough, I put it through the blender and applied it to the sores (as a poultice). To make a long story short, the ulcers filled in level and healed with no need for any skin graft. It was a godsend!"

A man we'll call Mr. O'D. suffered from diabetes and a leg ulcer that would not heal. He had tried cortisone and other antibiotic ointments. Finally, after many months, he tried placing a fresh clean okra leaf on his leg ulcer, three times a day for two weeks, then twice a day for another two weeks. During the last two weeks, a thin slice of onion was placed upon the okra leaf and bandaged in place. This healed it, where all else had failed.

Horribly Spotted Faces Clear!

Alma W., 79, besides being crippled with arthritis, was afflicted with an ugly, red, nipple-shaped growth on her nose, which was removed, but returned again. Finally, to relieve it, comfrey-root poultices were applied day and night. Almost immediately the inflammation disappeared. Soon the wart disappeared too, without a trace! And with the herbal remedies, her arthritic misery vanished!

A startling case was a woman with hundreds of ugly black warts covering her face, neck, and chest. She also had a paralysis of one side of her mouth. Her doctor, making no promises, told her about a raw juice therapy involving cabbage juice. In a few weeks, the ugly mess cleared almost completely and the paralysis disappeared!

Miss L.E. reports: "I had a very bad infection on my face, which no drug would help. I went to eight different doctors 37 times last year. All the treatments they gave me made my face worse. I started taking vitamin A every day and in three days the infection which I had for a year was clearing. Now my face looks wonderful."

Mrs. C.N. reports: "Recently I heard of zinc as a help for acne sufferers, and decided to try it. It works wonders. My skin, always loaded with blemishes, has never looked clearer. Believe it or not, I had acne into my thirties! No amount of scrubbing or lotions has ever done what zinc supplements accomplished in one short week."

Mrs. M.I. had been suffering for 25 years with large red, blotchy, scaly areas all over her face and neck. This ugly skin condition is called seborrhea, and the itching is intolerable. Four dermatologists had told her that this extremely uncomfortable and disfiguring condition could not be cured. "All prescribed creams and ointments for my skin," she says. "None of them really did much good at all.... I asked if it was some kind of vitamin deficiency. Each doctor said it was not. What could I say? They were the doctors." Then she heard about vitamin B-6 ointment for seborrhea, and got some. "It helped both the itching and redness more than the prescriptions I was using," she says. She also tried B-6 tablets. With 150 mg., "Wonderful things happened. Within days I could see results. Now, two weeks later, my face is almost completely healed."

Immediate Relief For Ingrown Toenails!

An article in *Lancet*, August 16, 1975, refers to "the almost savage practices generally employed in the cure" of ingrown toenails by doctors. Most suggested methods—which can only be done by doctors—seem dangerous, painful, and ineffective, with an admitted failure-rate of 64 percent! If you're still stuck with a thick, ugly, yellowish nail curling hideously deep into the skin, in a scroll-like fashion, you might try this simple method:

> "Having suffered severely from ingrown toenails for over 20 years, I was willing to try almost anything," says Mr. K.N. Then he heard about vitamin E for ingrown toenails. "I have faithfully applied vitamin E directly from a 200 I.U. capsule once each month for the past year," he says, "and I no longer have ingrown nails, nor have I the agony of periodically digging out the nail! I experienced immediate relief after the first application and have no recurrence whatsoever. I don't know why it works, but it does!"

Miss D.F. reports doing this, and her nail miraculously straightened and became normal again. She says: "Twenty years ago I got a fungus under the nail of my big toe. It pained occasionally and then it began to separate from the skin, and it soon humped across my toe, not flat and smooth like normal. I could not wear closed toe shoes for any length of time as the pressure on that raised nail made my toe sore. After hearing about vitamin E, I decided to try it. I began dropping vitamin E oil under the nail every day for several weeks, and I started to notice a nice healthy color in the nail (not the hard brittle look it had). Well, it took almost a year, but today that nail has completely attached itself to my toe and now is as flat and pretty as any normal nail."

Immediate Relief For Painful Toenails!

Mrs. A.H. reports: "Several years ago I developed a fungus infection under several toenails. The nails turned black and oozed, with a dreadful thickening of the flesh. Several nails fell off. I couldn't stand the pressure of any closed shoes. I tried every medicine a doctor gave me. All failed. Then I heard about vitamin E. Every night for two weeks I squeezed the oil from several capsules (400 I.U. each) on my toes. The results were nothing short of miraculous! The oozing stopped, the thick skin fell away and now my feet look attractive. My husband saw it, and is a witness to this miracle!"

Painful Sliver Of Wood Under Fingernail Gone!

Mrs. M.C. reports: "I had an agonizing infection from a redwood sliver under my fingernail. It was impossible to remove it and the finger was badly swollen and painful. I took a slice of onion and taped it around the area and overnight, swelling, plus sliver had disappeared completely!

Ms. R.J. reports: "I have had soft nails which break very easily. I tried many preparations to harden them, but nothing kept them hard for more than a couple of days. I started eating sunflower seeds every day after lunch, and after about two weeks I found my nails to be extra strong and staying that way. I have passed on this tip to several friends and they also find their nails are stronger than ever.

Mrs. S.N. reports: "All my life I'd had good fingernails, but about 10 years ago (at age 50) I began having trouble. My nails would 'peel' off in layers. They were so brittle, too, and would break easily. Three or four years of gelatin capsules and drugstore medicines were to no avail. Then a stranger said to me, 'Use dolomite!' I began with three tablets a day, plus a cod-liver oil tablet. I take bone meal, too. In less than three months my nails were strong and flexible again! After three years, I am convinced it is permanent."

Terrible Bedsores Vanish—Surgeon's Knife Avoided!

The medieval practice of removing bedsores by slicing them away with a knife is, unfortunately, still practiced by doctors. The procedure is called "debriding," and it must be done every day, if the sores are large and gangrenous.

It is excruciatingly painful, because an anesthetic cannot be used. The only way the doctor can tell if he has cut away all the dead, gangrenous tissue is by slicing deep

into healthy flesh. If the patient screams in pain, the dead flesh is gone.

A nurse reports using ordinary liquid lecithin—purchased at a local health food store—to heal two bedsores on the lower spine of a gentleman patient at the hospital where she worked. Three times a day the sores were cleansed with hydrogen peroxide, coated with liquid lecithin, and bandaged with a non-stick dressing. The patient did not lean on the sore area. In two days, everyone was surprised to find that the bedsores were healing nicely![1]

Incurable Vitiligo Cured!

Mrs. C.H. reports: "No cure for vitiligo? Don't you believe it, for I've found a cure so simple and pure it could be eaten. Not only did it work on me, but on all who have tried it. After having severe vitiligo and being to several doctors, all of whom told me there was no cure, I started studying vitiligo, its onset, its patterns, etc. After watching it spread, checking with others who had it, looking at it under a lens, I decided that something (probably detergents or soap) was destroying the acid mantle without which there can be no healthy skin.

"I made an acid mantle cream and, would you believe, in a week one could see a change in the color of the skin! From then on it was a steady climb back to a healthy skin without unsightly white patches.

"A well-known beauty expert says that pure mayonnaise is an almost perfect acid mantle. Crush five 100 mg. PABA tablets (this screens out harmful sun rays), dissolve in a quarter of a cup of hot (not boiling) water, and place in jar with a cup of pure mayonnaise. Shake well, and you've your per-

---

[1]In *Lancet*, September 7, 1974, T.V. Taylor, of Manchester Royal Infirmary reports that a group of geriatric patients were given 500 mg. of vitamin C twice daily, and in one month showed an average reduction in bedsores of 84 percent.

fect acid mantle. Use often, after every washing of hands or body. Desired results should be achieved in four to five months, depending upon the severity of the vitiligo."

A Miracle Medicine Food For Eczema!

Reportedly, eating raw potatoes has worked miracles in curing eczema and other skin eruptions. In one case, a young woman we'll call Miss J.A. had been suffering from a severe case of eczema since childhood. She was spending as much as $25 a week for drugstore preparations, which gave her some relief but did not cure the condition. An old lady told her about eating raw potatoes. She stopped taking drugs, and after a few weeks on the raw potato diet, her face cleared up. She continues eating one raw potato a day!

Poison Ivy Disappears —In Five Minutes!

A young man I knew, J.S., accidentally sat in some poison ivy. His entire body broke out in a massive inflammation, with itching that could only be relieved by soaking in a tub. A doctor told him to use expensive ointments, which helped little because they made his skin more alkaline (one gave him "cortisone bumps" on his fingers and caused a serious relapse).

> **Then he remembered reading that lemon juice is valuable in many skin conditions, such as acne, eczema, erysipelas, boils, carbuncles, blackheads, dandruff, sore and reddened hands—and that it will relieve the itch of insect bites, as well as irritation caused by poison oak or ivy. He sliced open a couple of lemons and rubbed them all over his body. In less than five minutes, his skin looked completely normal, and he felt immediate relief!**

The next day, his skin completely clear, he came to work —and accidentally reinfected his hands with items he had touched previously. The itching broke out again, his hands became raw, inflamed and lumpy. I told him to try washing with a vitamin C tablet, dissolved in water—but as no one had one, I suggested an orange that someone had brought for lunch. J.S. sliced the orange and rubbed it on his arms and hands. In less than five minutes, his skin looked completely normal!

Miracle Medicine Foods For Poison Oak!

Mrs. E.M. reports: "For three weeks I lived a miserable life of sleepless nights, and had such a distorted appearance that I vowed never to utter a complaint if I could just look like myself again. This was during a severe case of poison oak, covering my entire body, including eyes and ears. Then I found a remedy.

"Goldenseal, taken both internally and as a bath, performed a miracle. Twenty minutes after my first internal dose, the itching stopped and then I made a wash. The healing could practically be seen immediately.

"I used a quarter of a teaspoon per cup of hot water to drink and a teaspoon to a pint of hot water as a wash. I drank it about six times a day and washed very often. It is very bitter, so for those who cannot drink it, it can be put in blank capsules without any unpleasantness. I have continued drinking a cup or two daily and it has also acted as a preventative."

Ms. A.L. reports: "I am extremely allergic to poison oak which surrounds us here and which is almost impossible to eradicate. From time to time, I suffer dreadful attacks and then I have to take action. Before, when I was desperate, I broke down and had cortisone shots. Now, twice I have taken really massive doses of brewer's yeast, with warm water and honey to make it palatable as well as for their healing effects, and I devour this four, five, even up to seven times daily until I note the drying up process starting. This is usually noticeable by the end of one day. For anyone who suffers from this curse, I am sure they will not think this cure too drastic to try!"

Amazing Tea Relieves Cold Sores!

Mrs. L.V. reports: "I've been troubled with these 'horrid' things for years, and have recently been told of an old, old remedy. It really *works* and is so simple (even more so than yogurt) that it is not a health hazard in the least.

"I make a cup of sage tea, using two or three leaves of sage in a cup of water. When it is properly steeped I add one teaspoon of powdered ginger. It relieves my poor sore mouth and uptight stomach. I first began this treatment several years ago when I had five cold sores at a time.

"I drank several cups of the sage tea at intervals until they had disappeared (possibly three cups of tea). I had not had a recurrence until several weeks ago. I promptly took to my soothing cup of tea. Overnight the sores disappeared. It seems too simple to work, but it does, when all else fails."

Garlic Cures Impetigo!

Miss L.D. reports: "Within a year's time, infectious impetigo has victimized me twice. The first time, not knowing what it was and fearing its rapid spread and the unbearable itching, I went to the doctor. After two weeks of sticky medication, agonizing self-denial of scratching, and a $16 medical bill, I was finally relieved. I was satisfied to pay anything just to be relieved of the constant itching and the spreading of more itching that always followed.

"But this second time it all happened quite differently. One day, when my hands and face were to the point where I felt I had to see a doctor for medication... all of a sudden I realized that garlic might relieve the itching, if not cure the impetigo altogether. So I took one of my friend's pills, opened it, spread some garlic on the irritated areas and swallowed the remaining garlic. In half an hour, the itching was gone completely! I was able to sleep at night. I continued to rub fresh garlic on these areas and to eat garlic as long as it was necessary (three days)."

Garlic Oil Heals Blisters!

Mr. R.F. states: "I am a letter carrier and had suffered in pain from blisters that had developed from ill-fitting shoes. I had tried every pharmaceutical product on the market with absolutely no lessening in pain or size of the blisters.

"I then remembered the antiseptic properties of garlic and immediately rushed to the health food store and purchased a bottle of natural garlic perles. I broke open a few capsules and massaged the oil into my blistered feet. The next day the swellings were practically gone and no more pain!

"When I told this to my doctor he was dumbfounded! He could not believe that all the sophisticated medicines I had purchased from the drugstore had no effect on my blisters, while nature's simple garlic had ended my misery. I then threw all the unnatural drugs down my sink and vowed to trust Mother Nature first."

Garlic Vanquished Bedsores!

"Garlic is a sure cure for bedsores," says Mr. and Mrs. C.R.G.: "It is a miracle. I've tried everything that was recommended by nurses, hospitals and others, but nothing helped for nearly a year. . . . I read that garlic was good for boils and suppurating sores. So I tried it.

"I grated some garlic on a very fine grater, mixed it with oil, made a poultice to put over the bedsore, and left it on for two days. My husband said it burned. I was afraid to look at it. When I took the pad off, I couldn't believe my eyes. The scab was off, the swelling was down and there was no bleeding. Then I kept putting a pad with comfrey salve on it for over a week. All of the dead skin from around where the opening was peeled off. It was all smooth."

Painful Growths and Spastic Colon Healed!

M.V., a dentist, reports that for ten years he underwent X-ray and radium treatments to eradicate ugly skin growths that kept reappearing, even though a doctor said they were nonmalignant. On applying the juice of this amazing plant, garlic—which had relieved his spastic colon—the painful growths on his face completely disappeared!

> The first time he tried this was for a growth near his eye. He applied garlic oil—from capsules—regularly, and in about a month it disappeared! The next time he tried it was for a growth just inside his hair line which grew rapidly, in fact it was about the size of a nickle before he realized it was there. Again, apparently, garlic oil healed it!

These growths, he says, were caused by a severe sunburn, and the radiologist who diagnosed them advised him to use alcohol to dry them up—which he tried for two or three months without success. "Can you wonder," he says, "that we are interested in statements about garlic and cancer? Whether or not these growths were malignant, they certainly could have so developed, with my past history. And they were definitely not healing until we applied the garlic. Furthermore, they were unsightly and painful. We hope this experience of ours may prove helpful to others. The treatment is harmless and in our case proved most beneficial."

Garlic Cures Athlete's Foot!

For years, James T. suffered in silent misery from a "galloping case of athlete's foot," as he described it. He moaned that it was all due to a ringworm or fungus he picked up on a wet locker room floor. His toes were red, peeling, and painful. The heel and ball of his feet were rough with a million little dry pockmarks.

> He tried everything to get rid of it: frequent soaking, with soap and water, fresh dry stockings, powders, A&D ointment, antifungal creams. Some made it worse. Some actually did clear it up temporarily, but it would always come back, and the redness or peeling of the toes never really subsided. It was endless. His feet had an offensive

odor, and he was embarrassed to take his shoes off. There was burning, itching, and soreness.

In my experience—when all medicines have failed to help—garlic is a sure cure for athlete's foot. The method here is to spread some freshly crushed garlic over the affected area. It will feel warm for about five minutes. This should remain on the skin for a half hour. Then wash the foot with plain water. Do this once a day for a week, and goodbye, athlete's foot. (If the skin burns, remove the garlic immediately, wash with plain water, and try again later with diluted garlic juice mixed with water, until you find a mixture that doesn't burn, since too much garlic can worsen this condition.) To prevent reinfection, boil your socks.

Garlic Remedies For Acne

In *Of Men and Plants,* Maurice Mességué claims 90 percent cures for eczema and related skin problems, such as dermatosis and acne. These he divides into categories, such as acne of gastric (stomach) origin, and acne of intestinal origin. Here are two of these remedies—involving garlic.[2]

ACNE OF GASTRIC (STOMACH) ORIGIN
  Garlic (one large crushed head)
  Great burdock (leaves—one handful)
  Roman chamomile (one dozen crushed heads)
  Greater celandine (leaves, semi-fresh if possible—one handful)
  Peppermint (leaves—one handful)
  Nettle (leaves, fresh if possible—one handful)
  Thyme (leaves—one handful)

Make the basic preparation, following instructions on page 37, Chapter 2. Use this mixture for foot- and hand-

---

[2] Reprinted with permission of Macmillan Publishing Co., Inc., from *Of Men and Plants* by Maurice Mességué. Copyright © 1972 by Weidenfeld & Nicolson Ltd. Copyright © 1973 by Macmillan Publishing Co., Inc.,

baths, he says, or by pouring it over a poultice made from cabbage and watercress, as described in Chapter 4, page 78—and applying to the stomach. It is not to be eaten or taken internally.

> **ACNE OF INTESTINAL ORIGIN**
> Garlic (one large crushed head)
> Great burdock (flowers and leaves—one handful)
> Roman chamomile (one dozen crushed heads)
> Greater celandine (leaves and flowers, semi-fresh if possible—one handful)
> Field bindweed (flowers—one handful)
> Round-leaved mallow (flowers—one handful)

To make this basic preparation, follow instructions on page 37, Chapter 2, and use in foot- and hand-baths. Or make a poultice, following instructions on page 78, Chapter 4, using cabbage and fresh nettle leaves, to be coated with a liqueur glass of the basic preparation and applied to the stomach. Do not eat or drink.

Mességué states that while these remedies can bring relief, they are not necessarily a cure, since acne can be due to many different conditions—liver, bowel, or stomach trouble, or change of life. For all skin diseases, he advises, follow the diet prescribed by a doctor.

Skin Eruptions On Face Cured!

Amanda B., a college girl, knew she had a bad stomach (she was always complaining of heartburn and indigestion). But her biggest problem, it seemed, was ugly, unsightly acne all over her forehead, her cheeks, and even her jaw. Large pink pustules were forever forming, she said—no matter how carefully she cleansed her face.

The itching was sometimes uncontrollable, and scratching only made it worse. Ugly scabs formed. She had been to a doctor, she said, and used lotions and antibiotics. Nothing seemed to help. Careful dieting had been suggested to eliminate certain foods—such as sweets—that might be

aggravating the situation. But Amanda couldn't resist an occasional malted milk or chocolate bar.

No one could suggest eating garlic to her, to detoxify her system. She would never hear of it. But someone did suggest Mességué's external applications, which she agreed to try. Lo and behold! The acne cleared up—the pustules faded and decreased in number—and her face became healthy and smooth.

Onion For Snakebite and Stings!

In 1897, Dr. Fernie wrote in his book, *Herbal Simples:* "The juice of a sliced raw onion is alkaline, and will quickly relieve the acid venom of a sting from a wasp or bee, if applied immediately to the parts...."

In 1972, this bit of advice came in handy for a young lady who wrote: "Two years ago while riding my motorcycle, I got a yellow jacket in between my little toe and the one next to it. By the time I was able to park my bike, I got stung badly. I was over 75 miles from home, but I finally made it. When I got in the house I tried everything imaginable. Finally, I remembered my grandmother putting an onion on a sting I had as a little girl.

"By now," says this writer, who we'll call Miss A.V., "my foot was three times its normal size, but I tried it anyway. In less than thirty minutes my foot was back to normal, and never even knew it had been stung. When I went to work the next day I told several of my customers about my experience. Most of them listened but none really believed me."[3]

Honey Relieves Hornet Stings!

Mrs. A.W. reports: "My husband was mowing the lawn, dressed in shorts, when a swarm of hornets attacked him. He

---

[3] For snakebites, an old-time method settlers used was to crush some onion, mix in a few drops of kerosene, and apply this in a poultice to the affected area. It was said that this poultice "draws out the poison as is seen by the green color of the poultice after it has been on the bite for a short time."

dashed into the house and rolled on the floor to dislodge some hornets that were still biting him, and screamed for a doctor. I frantically started dabbing honey all over his legs and arms. The honey started to relieve his terrible pains almost immediately! (My sister who told me this secret said to alternate honey with ice bags.) And the wonderful part of it is that he had hardly any swelling!" Instant pain relief!

Wheat Germ Oil For Stings!

Mrs. M.G. reports: "Wheat germ oil is a sure cure for stings. Last summer a wasp stung my brother. He decided to try wheat germ oil and discovered it relieved all pain as soon as it was applied. Hornets stung my arm and hand. I rubbed wheat germ oil on and instantly the pain left—no swelling. Try it. It is a miracle how quickly it relieves and cures stings. It is also good for frostbite and chapped hands and fever blisters."

Miracle Medicine Foods
For Canker Sores!

Mrs. L.C. reports: "A problem I had for quite a few years was frequent and very painful canker sores. I would scarcely get over one and another would start. A chiropractor friend suggested that I take vitamin B-2 (riboflavin) and see if it would help. After I started to take the B-2, the cankers became much less frequent and of shorter duration. I now very seldom have one and if one ever does come it usually doesn't last very long. (There's very little discomfort.)"

Mrs. M.M. reports: "My ten-year-old son was plagued for months with canker sores—one right after another—sometimes three at a time. Then I was told this herpes simplex virus responded very well to the bacteria in yogurt known as lactobacillus acidophilus.

"Not caring for yogurt, my son prefers taking the tablets that are available through most of the companies selling natural vitamins. I started him off taking two at each meal. Within three days the canker sores were almost gone—the pain left sooner than that. I gradually decreased the number of daily tablets and now give them at the first sign of a canker sore. Not only is he much relieved, but other members of our family who suffer from cold sores, fever blisters, and canker sores have much less of a problem. I couldn't help bragging to our doctor about my 'find,' and he told me he's prescribing 'lacto' to his patients with this stubborn problem."

A Horrible Case Of Vitiligo Healing Miraculously!

Mrs. A.W. reports: "One day I was surprised to discover white patches on the inside of my wrists. (These patches were about the size of a fifty-cent piece.) In time these ugly splotches had spread into the areas of my thumbs and hands. I was 32 years of age when I first detected the first signs of this skin disease called vitiligo or leukoderma.

"As the years passed, these splotches, or loss of pigment took over larger areas of my body until I was completely void of all pigmentation of the skin. During these years, I consulted many well-known dermatologists and other specialists, who in turn sent me to medical laboratories for various tests. Other doctors just frankly informed me that there wasn't anything that they could do to help me.

"It seemed I was destined to suffer this embarrassment the rest of my life. Fortunately for me, my husband had schooled himself by reading many books on nutrition. One evening he was reading about an English nutritionist who was proving himself to be successful in overcoming vitiligo by prescribing to his patients the vitamin B family in daily dosages. According to his writings, those with vitiligo were responding beautifully and they were actually regaining the pigmentation of their skin.

"About this time my husband discovered a bit of news that left us wide-eyed with wonder and amazement. My husband discovered that my symptoms of excruciating burning ... whenever I would reach out or lift any lightweight object

... could be a dangerous deficiency of the vitamin B family.

"I immediately started taking natural vitamin B food supplements plus other all-natural vitamins on a well-balanced high protein diet. Within ten days I felt less burning everywhere. As I continued my vitamin B intake, I began to notice with great excitement that I was regaining the pigment in my lower arms. My case was a bad one, but at this writing the natural pigmentation has formed small islands on my upper left arm from the wrist to the elbow. On the other arm these islands have fused from the wrist to the elbow and appear healthy and normal again. ..."

Another Miracle Food Heals Burns!

Mr. F.C. reports: "A young fellow next door was working on his hot rod when his shirt caught fire from flaming gasoline. My wife heard his screams and we ran out and ripped his shirt off. My wife poured apple cider vinegar on his back, and he said the pain was gone immediately. A fireman at the scene told her to stop, but the boy said, "Please don't." He was 17 years old. There was no more pain and no sign of scars.

"A young girl down the street burned the inside of her leg on the hot manifold of a Honda. She was screaming with pain until apple cider vinegar was splashed on, then looked up in amazement and said wonderingly, 'It doesn't hurt any more.' Again, no scar ever became evident.

"My wife splashed hot grease from a skillet on to her upper chest and neck. Immediately she splashed the apple cider vinegar on the affected areas. Result: No more pain or evidence of scars."

15

Miracle Medicine Foods For Arthritis!

"Several years ago," says Mrs. S.J., "I got terrible pains in my back and legs. I went to see a doctor who said I had a bad case of arthritis. He didn't need to tell me that! He sent me to another doctor for x-rays (I don't know why) who corroborated the diagnosis and also recommended a heating pad and pain-killing pills. No cure, both doctors said. I found a cure.

"Luckily, I had just read that you can cure arthritis by eating pecans, bananas, brewer's yeast, wheat germ, and avocados, plus anything else you want to eat. Well, why not try it? I did. In a few days I abandoned the pills and heating pad, and in less than two weeks there was no more pain at all and has never been any since. Great for cereals and desserts!

"I suppose the reason I didn't broadcast this was that I thought everyone would say: 'Oh, that couldn't have been arthritis.' But about nine months ago, the man who delivered my milk came down with arthritis so badly that his doctor told him he would have to quit his job, he couldn't drive a car any more. When I heard that I telephoned him at his home and told him my experience. He tried it, was back on the job in ten days, and is still on it, feeling fine.

Lady Cured Of Arthritis Wants To Tell The World Her Secret!

"Of course then I began to spread the good word. When friends come to see me, the first thing I ask them is: 'Do you know anyone who has arthritis?' The answer is always 'Yes,' and I tell my story. The postman brings me many letters with glowing reports of results. One woman in New Jersey sent me some avocados, in gratitude, because I had told her that I often couldn't get them.

"I have no reason to believe that I must keep on eating these things, but I like them, so I eat them now and then. One thing I like about this is that I have told it to six doctors, and every one of them got a pen and wrote down the short list of what one should eat. Wouldn't that make you feel good?"

Pain and Swelling Disappear In Ankles, Legs and Wrists!

Mrs. F.L. reports: "I never realized just how badly my ankles, wrists and fingers were swollen until my fingers began to have sharp fleeting pains, especially in the joints. This was of special concern to me as I am a typist, violinist, and stenographer. My hands are my livelihood.

> "Vitamin B complex drained off pounds of water; my fingers now look actually 'skinny' and the pains are completely gone. My ankles, legs, and wrists are much thinner, and the most important thing, my spirits have been lifted tremendously.

"I almost feel like I get a 'high' from B vitamins. (By the way, when I asked my doctor if I might have a B deficiency, he almost laughed at me.) Also, I noticed another effect—since taking the vitamins my monthly period has been cut almost in half. And another thing—my craving for sweets, which I have fought for years, has been diminished."

Excruciating Wrist Pain Gone!

Mrs. H.E. reports: "Last year, after spraining my wrist several times, I lost the use of it completely. A prescription for the pain did nothing for the wrist, and made me sleepy. Later, my doctor gave me a new prescription, assuring me that it wouldn't bother me. I developed mysterious stomach aches. The stomach problems disappeared a few weeks after quitting the second medication, but I still had the sore wrist.

"I am a writer, and I could not type five minutes without developing the most excruciating pain in my sore wrist. Even writing a check was painful. Then I heard about taking vitamin B-6 for stiffness, and started taking about 50 mg. daily. I got excellent results within a few weeks.

"Last week I put in six straight hours at my typewriter without a twinge! I might add that . . . this was the only new change in my diet." This woman had already been taking B complex, A,C,D and calcium. Only B-6 worked for her.

Painful Heel Spur Relieved!

Mrs. L.B. reports: "Several years ago, I suffered pain in my right heel every time I put the foot down. It was very painful. I consulted a general practitioner and was told I most likely had a heel spur. The doctor prescribed pills and ointment which did not bring any relief. After several visits, it was decided to have the heel x-rayed. Two days later the physician told me that it was a spur; he could not help nor could a specialist, just 'wear a soft pad in your shoe to ease the pain.'

"I was desperate. Only a person who has suffered a heel spur can know what that means. When I read press reports about vitamin C and arthritis, I bought some and started ingesting it at the rate of four or five grams per day. On the third day, the heel was not painful to lean on anymore—and only slightly when pressed hard with a finger.

"About a year later, I had the heel x-rayed again since the doctor and I were both curious to know what had happened. I thought the spur had dissolved, but the x-ray showed it was still there. A mystery!"

Shoulder Pain Vanishes Almost Immediately!

Mrs. E.L. reports: "I sprained my shoulder and was given aspirin and codeine for the excruciating pain that made it impossible to get more than two or three hours of sleep a night. The medicine was ineffective, and then I remembered reading about vitamin E for nerve and muscle pain. I decided to try it after experiencing the worst night I'd ever had with my shoulder pain. After the first treatment of vitamin E and calcium, I was pain-free. It was amazing, and a wonderful relief, because I have since been able to sleep from six to eight hours at night, pain-free!"

Knee Pain Disappeared!

Mr. B.E. reports: "I hardly believe what has happened! Several years ago I tore the ligaments in my knee and was on crutches off and on whenever I exercised. I went to New York to see a famous specialist who prescribed exercises with weights (and arch supports). After three years, the pain was still there.... Then I heard about the experience of others with knee pain and I started taking 600 to 800 I.U. of vitamin E. Within a week the pain disappeared."

Mrs. L.A. reports: "About one and a half years ago I was suffering with arthritis in my knee. My doctor recommended wearing a rubber stocking on the knee. This had no effect at all.... The pain was severe and I couldn't sleep at night. Walking was painfully difficult, even with a cane. Going up and down stairs was almost impossible.

"Then I began taking vitamin C, vitamin E, bone meal and dolomite. In about two weeks the pain was entirely gone, to my great joy and amazement! Gradually the stiffness disappeared, and in a month's time I was walking freely."

Crippling Leg Pain Gone!

Mr. A.E. reports: "I suffered with enough pain of an arthritic nature in my right lower limb to last ten lifetimes. The pain began gradually, slowly becoming unbearable in a few years. In order to walk, I needed a cane. I couldn't be without it. Sometimes I would lean on my wife's shoulder in order to navigate. Words cannot describe that excruciating pain.... The owner of a health food store noticed my cane, and suggested vitamin E. I was skeptical.

> **"Now here is where the miracle occurred. In three or four days, the pain in my leg lessened. I stopped the aspirin. In a week, I could walk without a cane or limp. The impossible had happened. Can you possibly imagine my relief? I had suffered for 14 years. I have not taken one aspirin in five years.**

"At the present time, on a doctor's advice, I take 400 I.U. at each meal. I have no pain whatsoever in my limb. To prove that it was not just my imagination that cured the pain, I stopped taking it twice. Both times, the pain returned with a vengeance. I am now fully convinced it is the vitamin E. Before this, my physician could only suggest aspirin."

Amazing New Miracle Medicine Foods Bring Fast Relief From Arthritic Agony!

"Unbelieveable—but true!" say grateful arthritis sufferers! All over America, arthritis sufferers are talking about a remarkable new way to get incredible relief from the agonies of painful arthritic joint inflammation and stiffness! Reportedly, amazing new miracle medicine foods give comforting relief, reduce aching joint inflammation and stop arthritic pain!

"What a difference! What a joy!" That's what arthritic sufferers are saying. Tested and proven by thousands of users—in scores of documented reports—ALL enthusiastically agreed these miracle rejuvenation foods give faster, more effective relief than they ever got before—all-day, all-night relief that seems permanent! Here are anesthetic healing foods said to make pain vanish, often in a matter of minutes!

Arthritic Back In Wonderful Shape Now, Thanks To Alfalfa Tea!

Mr. H.N. reports: "I have had arthritis in my back for a number of years. Three months ago it was so bad I could hardly get in and out of my car. Then I learned of a woman who had cured her arthritis by drinking alfalfa tea. I decided to try alfalfa seeds for my problem. I grind up three tablespoons every day and mix with yogurt or milk as part of my lunch. I am delighted that my back is in wonderful shape again."

> Mrs. A.Y. reports: "I have personally experienced a miracle in my life. For nine years I suffered with rheumatoid arthritis—I lived on aspirins, then cortisone, Indocin, Butazolidin, etc. but not one of these helped. My heart problems were innumerable and I had quite a bit of crippling from the arthritis.

"My weight went down to 96 pounds (I'm five feet nine). I was anemic, my white cell count was abnormal and, worst of all, I was in constant severe pain. Then a friend recommended alfalfa tea (an ounce of alfalfa seed in hot but not boiling water—a little over half a quart—simmered for 30 minutes, strained, cooled and refrigerated not longer than 24 hours, as beverage with water, half-and-half, or honey to taste, for four or five times a day or more).

"I began drinking it every day for about three months (and now at least twice a week). My health improved and the pain lessened every day. Today I live a nearly normal life, my blood count is normal, and my weight is 140 pounds. To the best of my ability, I avoid sugar, coffee, chemicals, overly processed foods, and white flour, but include fresh fruits and vegetables, vitamins, bran, and eat less meat and more non-meat protein. Every day I thank God that my life has turned around from a bed-ridden cripple to a useful contributing citizen."

Cherry Juice For Arthritis!

Cherries may bring you amazing relief from arthritis—without drugs. All-day, all-night relief that seems permanent, in many cases. Ludwig W. Blau, M.D., in *Texas Reports on Biology and Medicine* (volume 8) tells of an astounding cure among arthritis patients who were given cherry juice.

> Twelve gout patients were remarkably relieved by taking cherry juice. The report says that "no attacks of gouty arthritis have occurred on a nonrestricted diet in all 12 cases, as a result of eating about one-half pound of fresh or canned cherries per day."

This amazing fruit, often used in ice cream, cake, candy and desserts, may relieve your arthritis! Dr. Blau tells of astonishing cures by eating cherries—canned, sour, black, Royal Anne, or fresh black Bing cherries. One arthritis patient just drank the juice and the curative powers were equally effective.

Reported Cases:
- Dr. S.T. reports: "A patient of mine had heard about cherries for gout. He was, in fact, a sufferer of gout himself. He decided to give the cherry therapy a try. After following this patient's progress over the past two months, I can only say the results have been nothing less than spectacular. The patient has ceased taking the prescribed medication for his gout and has an unlimited diet. This alone should make any gout sufferer take notice. It can't do any harm to try it."
- Mrs. A.L. reports: "I am writing to tell you of my amazing relief from arthritis more than ten years ago. I had bought some sour cherries to make a pie, but sat around picking at them until I had eaten about a pound of them. Within a few hours, pain had left my shoulder

and arm. I continued eating the sour cherries during their season and had relief the entire time. When I stopped eating them, the pain returned. I usually freeze cherries every year for pies, but instead of making pies, I resumed eating my frozen cherries. Doctors, family and lay people as well all laughed at me, but I still maintain that cherries were my cure for arthritis. Since that time if I ever get an attack I head for the freezer and my cherries."

- Mrs. M.G. reports: "After hearing about them, I began eating red, sour cherries for my gout. I had been taking various drugs, but I still had a lot of swelling. By eating the cherries daily, I have been able to leave off medications entirely, and the swelling in my ankles is gone. By adding vitamin E to my diet, the terrible leg pains I was plagued with at night have been greatly reduced also. Through the use of vitamins and food supplements, I have been able to stop using all arthritis medications. This is the first time in 20 years that I have been able to leave off drugs for arthritis."

- Mrs. R.I. reports: "I have suffered with an aching, throbbing knee for almost two years. After going to several doctors and chiropractors, having knee x-rays and taking bottles of aspirin, I was about to give up. With two children and many years ahead of me (I'm 29) I had to find something. By accident one day I heard about cherries for gout.... I had gout, so after hearing this, I immediately bought several cans of cherries. I ate them for about a week, and all the swelling and stiffness disappeared! It was a miracle! As long as I eat cherries, there is no pain. Exercise, walking, bicycling and no pain.... I will eat cherries the rest of my life—they are fantastic!"

- Mrs. E.N. reports: "I am 62 years old, in excellent health, and have never had an operation. But I do have arthritic fingers. After hearing about cherries for gout, I started eating cherries and drinking cherry juice; and I haven't stopped yet. After two weeks there was a noticeable improvement in my fingers—the swelling was

less; the pain was gone. I hadn't been able to make a fist, and now I can. When cherries were in season, I froze 24 pounds, and just ran out of them yesterday. However, I will continue to drink cherry juice and eat canned cherries until the cherry season is here next year. Life *can* be a bowl of cherries!"
- Mrs. A.N. reports: "I started eating cherries about a month and a half ago. After about a week I woke up one morning and felt like a new person. My skin was clear, swelling was gone and I could bend my fingers completely and painlessly. My wrists and ankles shrank, I wasn't even aware they were swollen before. Painful years of suffering and shame of unsightly splits and sometimes bleeding hands were gone. I couldn't believe it."

Bone Meal Relieves Bone Aches!

"About four years ago," says Ms. M.A., "I started to develop arthritis. I consulted six doctors, and was given several reasons for it, but no help. Most seemed to agree the only thing was to 'learn to live with it.' I tried but at times it seemed the marrow in my bones had a toothache.

"At times I could not even turn a water faucet on. I prayed until I think even God must have tired of me. I would lie on the bed and say, 'Today, God, I hurt in my ankle, my arm and my thumb.' The prayer seemed to help. And then one day I heard that bone meal was good for 'bone aches.' I got a bottle and started taking six to nine tablets a day. . . .

"I know three months does not make a cure, but I no longer have pains. I can move now easily and I am off pain-killing drugs. I used to use about 200 Arthritis Pain Formula pills ever five or six weeks. Now I do not take any at all . . . My husband suggested we give some bone meal to our dog, and she also has lost her limp."

Knee Pain Relived By Apple Cider Vinegar!

Mrs. A.T. reports: "My father had a bad knee from kneeling on cement welding for 20 years. A couple of years ago it started getting so bad he would miss work and have to stay home with a heating pad on it. The knee would swell to twice its normal size.

"On one occasion, his knee completely gave out crossing a street and he collapsed on the ground. He had gone to doctors about it and they found nothing. They gave him pain killers but nothing helped.

"About a year ago my brother, who is very health conscious, had him drink one part apple cider vinegar to two parts water every day. After a couple of weeks, the pain subsided. Eventually the pain and swelling completely left and didn't return." (As long as he kept drinking this mixture.)

Herbal Bath Completely Relieves Painful Feet and Legs!

Mrs. E.L. reports: "After reading the book *Of Men and Plants*, the autobiography of the Frenchman, Mességué, who heals people with herbs, I decided to try one of the foot baths he recommends. I had been having severe pains in my legs for several weeks; my legs became tired after only a few blocks of walking. He recommends a mixture of about seven or eight different herbs.... I used just what I had on hand... which was a large quantity of elderberry tea, and a mixture of about ten herbs in an herbal tea containing camomile, dock, peppermint, oat straw, horsetail, linden blossom, red clover, alfalfa, fennel seed, and rose hips. After boiling the water, I put the herbs in—about two tablespoons of elderberry and two of the mixture—boiled it and then steeped it, simmeringly gently on the fire for about 15 minutes.

"Then I put the brew in a pan and bathed my feet in it ... Oh! what a comforting relief it was! Immediately, I felt a wonderfully refreshing feeling coursing through my legs, and my legs and feet began to tingle ... When I took my feet out about ten minutes later, the pains were completely gone and they felt so strong and new! It was really amazing.

"The next day, the pain was still gone, and the feeling of strength was still there.... The foot baths seem to affect not just the feet and legs, but the whole body. I feel much more energetic and rejuvenated since taking the foot baths. I hope this story will help someone."

Sea Water, Aging and Arthritis!

The sea is an inexhaustible reservoir of valuable minerals for arthritis sufferers. Sea water contains every known trace element, plus innumerable elements that have yet to be discovered. Apparently, to be healthy, we need the minerals sea water contains. Of course, not all sea water is good to drink. The kind sold in health food stores is germ free. In one miraculous case—

> Kenneth D., 92, was senile and completely crippled with arthritis. He had to be lifted out of bed and could not feed or dress himself. On a doctor's advice, he was given one teaspoonful of concentrated sea water per day. Suddenly he began to perk up. He got out of bed one day, hobbled into the kitchen, and began fixing breakfast!

After being senile and crippled for many years, he began to get up every morning without help and put on his clothes. Then he'd walk to the bathroom, wash, and come in for breakfast. His doctor reports he'd had an arthritic hip for over 20 years, and would yell if anyone touched his right leg even gently. But now he crossed his legs to put his shoes on, and let the right foot hit the floor without a peep. Reportedly, the only new item in his food or drink was the daily teaspoonful of sea water, the kind sold in health food stores, concentrated to ten times the usual ocean strength.

Liver and Arthritis!

Mr. G.D. reports: "Eight months ago I bought some dessicated liver, never dreaming it would really do wonders for my health. ... I am 53 and my health was failing fast. I had arthritis of the spine in an advanced stage (due to some bad falls I had).... But I kept reading, praying and searching, until one day God guided me to the health food store.

"In three days after taking four a day, I could jump out of bed without dragging myself.... My friends who had not seen me for months could hardly believe I was the same person they once knew. And do you think I tell them what I have discovered? You bet I do!

"I have started over 50 people taking dessicated liver. This is what it has done for me. No pain any more, no nausea, nerves calm, no colitis, no phlegm in my throat, and my headaches have stopped."

Olive Oil and Bursitis!

In one reported case, Mrs. R.B. says: "My husband had arthritis for seven years and at one time got a bad case of bursitis in his right shoulder and was unable to raise his arm. To relieve the soreness I started massaging the shoulder and upper arm daily with hot olive oil, using slight manipulation while massaging. This helped and gradually he got the motion back in his shoulder and hasn't been bothered with bursitis since."

Honey and Arthritis!

The story is told of a schoolteacher who had long been afflicted with arthritis and who had reached the point where she felt she just had to "live with it." She moved to a boarding house, where honey was served instead of sugar. Within a short time, she found—to her amazement—that her arthritis had disappeared!

A Swiss doctor reports the case of a man whose finger was smashed in a grinding machine. The bone at the tip of the finger was broken and hung by a flap of skin. After wrapping the finger in honey, it grew on and rapidly healed!

Vitamin C Helped Her Back Pain!

Ms. R.L. reports: "I want everyone to know what vitamin C has done for me. To begin with, my back began to bother me about six months ago. I'd never had back trouble in my entire life. It was so bad, I went to two back specialists. I was told I was born with a crooked bone next to my spine. I was given exercises and muscle relaxers to take four times a day.

"Well, the pills were like drinking water and the exercises made it worse. I gave up in tears. Then three months later, I heard about vitamin C for bad backs. I began on 2,000 mg. of vitamin C. I must admit I was skeptical at first, but my soreness disappeared in two days. Hallelujah!

"I stayed on 2,000 mg. a day and I started a vigorous exercise program of one hour every day. I have yet to feel the first pain or stiff or sore muscle. I couldn't even get out of bed three months ago."[1]

---

[1] An expert on vitamin C therapy, Dr. James Greenwood—himself a victim of low back and hip pain—recommends 500 mg. with every meal to patients with all kinds of ligament, back, hip, neck and arm pain. He says that pain disappears in 24 to 48 hours, and say that 93 percent have had dramatic relief and are able to do heavy work, including hiking and tennis. He adds that a large number with disc lesions were able to avoid surgery, and that this will eliminate most common back pains, sprains and disc ruptures. He says that exercise is necessary to help the vitamin reach all parts of the spine. (Caution: large doses of vitamin C—7,000 to 8,000 mg. —taken all at once, especially on an empty stomach, could cause abnormal cell growth, says a medical expert. Smaller amounts are not harmful, he says.)

Disc Slips Back In Place!

Mr. J.N. reports: "I was riding in the back of a truck in World War II when the driver lost control . . . and rolled us into a ditch. I ended up with a fractured fifth cervical and displacement (slipped disc). The Veterans' Administration told me I would never be any better, and might even get worse. . . . My symptoms included stiff neck muscles, headache, several vertebrae misaligned, sore muscles under tension. . . . After several years I noticed that when I had a cold I never had anything wrong with my back. . . . Then I realized it must be the vitamin C I was taking.

"The next time my neck started to tighten up I took a gram of vitamin C in the morning and another gram at night. The neck muscles loosened up, and the vertebrae creaked and cracked, going back in place, and I had no more pain. For the last five years I have kept myself free of back pain by taking twice my normal amount of vitamin C every time my neck starts to tighten up. . . .

"Vitamin C alone is not the cure. I try to take a complete complement of vitamins both as natural foods and supplements, but the addition of large doses of vitamin C seems to be specific for washing the bad guys out of my system. These are the results of 20 years of practical experience."

Bioflavonoids and Bursitis!

"I'm a hairdresser," says Mrs. V.L., "and use my arms a lot. I had bursitis in both arms. Several times I had to have cortisone injected into my shoulders, which was very painful, but the bursitis was more painful. When I heard about vitamin P (bioflavonoids) for bursitis, I bought tablets containing 400 mg. of C, 400 mg. of citric bioflavonoids and 50 mg. of rutin. I took three per day. Within two weeks, there was no more pain. That was three years ago. During that time I have been on a complete nutritional program. My doctor told me when I had been cured five years he would give the vitamins credit for it. I have shared this with others; they have had the same results."

Comfrey Poultice Healed Wrist!

Mrs. A.M. reports: "Some time ago I was suffering with pain in my wrist to the point where I could not write, use scissors, twist lids on or off jars, or do anything that caused pressure in my wrist. I had to work with my left hand as much as possible. I went to a doctor, and after x-rays and examinations, was told that it was either arthritis or synovitis —and no treatment was recommended.

"**I continued suffering with this wrist ailment for ten months. Then some friends, who were knowledgeable about comfrey, suggested that I try comfrey poultices. Fortunately, we had a sizeable patch in our garden. Every night for two weeks, my husband helped me prepare the comfrey and put it on my wrist.**

"We simply ground several leaves finely, then spread this mixture on a cloth, sometimes adding water if it seemed dry, and bound it around my wrist, covering it with plastic to keep from staining the sheets and taped it all together. In the morning we would would take it off. By the end of two weeks the pain was gone and we discontinued the treatment.

"More than a year has passed since my wrist recovered, and I have had no recurrence of the pain—nor have I had to use any more comfrey poultices."

Poke Berries For Arthritis!

An 83-year-old woman, Mrs. L.O. reports that poke berries are what keeps her arthritis in check, instead of the four tablets a day of aspirin that had been prescribed by a doctor. She takes three or four with each meal all year round, and keeps them in her refrigerator. The weed patch keeps her supplied. She says that others report the same amazing relief. "A proven remedy . . . it works!" she says.

Mrs. T.A. reports: "I can truthfully say that poke berries have helped my stiffness and blood pressure, and now I can sleep for six to eight hours every night whereas be-

fore I couldn't. When I went to see my doctor the other day, he wanted to know what I was doing. When I told him, he wrote it down and said the next time he went to a convention he would tell about it."

Poke weed grows mainly in the Eastern United States, as far north as Quebec and as far south as Mexico. Mrs. L.O. adds: "I let the poke grow in my back yard, but usually people pull it up as a weed. But they do gather the leaves in the spring to cook greens or to use as salads. It is not poisonous as many say. The roots may be, and a man who reported having taken three *dried* berries told of feeling sick afterward. I even heard of one lady who made pies with them.... The poke is not dried, but taken fresh and stored in plastic or glass containers in the refrigerator."

Another lady reports: "Poke is a springtime-only weed and it is poisonous later on in summer. The leaves and tender shoots can be canned the same as mustard or turnip greens. I put up two or three jars each spring."

Nerve Massage: Miracle Medicine Food for Arthritic Pain!

Regardless of where your pain is, massage both feet, completely, concentrating on any tender spots—which would indicate a nerve that leads to your troubled area. This painful area may be your arms, your back, or anywhere else —it doesn't matter. They can be soothed by rubbing the nerves that lead to them, starting in the feet, say experts. Do this once every other day.

For spinal troubles, massage along the inner edge of each foot, from toe to heel—for pain in the upper back, massage just below the big toe; for pain in the middle of the back, massage the center of the arch at the rim; for low back pain, massage along the inner edge near the heel.

Massage for at least a minute or two. If you wish you may use your hands. Massage both hands completely, especially in back of the thumbs, the pad at the base of the thumb, center of the palm, outer edge of wrist, pad along base of fingers, and between thumb and first finger. For low back pain, massage at the base of the thumb (top surface of hand). For pain in the center of the back, massage further up between wrist and web of thumb. For pain in upper back, shoulders or neck, massage the palm of the hand near base of thumb.

Reported Cases:
- Regardless of the cause of back pain, immediate relief almost always follows the use of this miracle medicine food—nerve massage—says one expert. Lumbago responds very quickly says one doctor. Patients straightened out almost immediately.
- This doctor tells of a case of backache that lasted for three months. Every form of treatment was tried without success. The man was bent almost double, unable to stand erect. With this miracle medicine food—nerve massage—in about 10 minutes, he straightened up, entirely relieved of pain. It works almost every time, says this doctor!
- A man unable to move without help, tried it, in 20 minutes, he was able to rise and walk, entirely relieved of pain!
- A man with a slipped disc was told by doctors he would only get worse unless he had an operation. His back frequently gave out without warning. With this secret, he was entirely relieved, has not had any trouble in years, and avoided surgery!

Foot Massage Relieves Back Pain!

Mrs. B.K. reports: "For years, I suffered low back pain and sciatica in my left leg. It became very bad while I was in college, and two years in a row I had to wear a full back brace. Sitting was practically impossible. An orthopedic surgeon found a flattened disk in my x-rays, and recommended exercise—which I did faithfully for seven years. The pain kept returning.

"About two years ago I became very interested in all forms of natural healing. I began to use foot massage. And this is the exciting part—it works! I have been able to control the pain in my back without exercises, the brace, or any special care in moving.

"As most foot charts will show, the nerves for the lower back run along the inside of the foot from the arch to the heel. Whenever I feel any pain in my back, I massage those nerves that are sore or tender for three or four minutes. If the pain continues as when I have strained my back by lifting something too heavy—like a bag of cement—I take two or three hot baths in a day and massage the nerves several times daily, for two or three days. The only precaution in massaging the nerves for the lower back is not to bruise the blood vessels by going too deeply. Generally, I massage as deeply as the tender reflex will allow."

Calcium For Pain Relief!

In his book, *An Eighty Year Old Doctor's Secrets of Positive Health* (Prentice-Hall, 1961), William Brady states: "Now it should be common knowledge yet it isn't even among doctors, that if one absorbs enough calcium from day to day, it will do for the body what analgesics, sedatives and narcotics only *seem* to do. Sedatives and narcotics are half-measures. Calcium is the real thing."

A Cure For Arthritis?

Dr. Brady, a medical doctor and syndicated writer whose health column was read by millions, defines all forms of arthritis as "rheumatiz", and says this method will relieve or cure them. He states:

"In the treatment of chronic joint disability—whether you prefer to call it arthritis or rheumatism—the so-called wonder drugs so lavishly prescribed by the merchants of medicine give no lasting benefit, but correction of the lifelong nutritional deficiencies which cause the disability usually give not only lasting benefits, but often also cures..."

"If you ask me about 'rheumatiz' I'll tell you it is degeneration of the joint tissues due to nutritional deficiency ... and that it is chiefly a calcium, vitamin D, iodine and vitamin B *deficiency. There is no more to tell about the nature and cause of insidiously developing joint disability of long standing..."* It's that simple, he says!

"The concept of chronic joint disability I present here is not something I picked out of the air. It is a conviction that came from a professional lifetime study of the question. I am not promoting any remedy or cure. I merely recommend a regimen, a way of life to prevent, relieve or, if adopted in time and consistently followed for life, perhaps even cure the 'rheumatiz'. This last claim I hesitate to make. But I am emboldened to speak of cure by numerous reports I have received from victims who declare they really are cured and back at their jobs their 'rheumatiz' forced them to give up."

Dr. Brady's Wonder Cure!

"The regimen is basically quite simple," says Dr. Brady. "The essential features are adequate daily rations of calcium, vitamin D, iodine and vitamin B complex." He says the best food sources for these are 1½ pints of milk, an ounce of cod liver oil, and plain wheat—daily! In addition, he says, you need an optimal daily ration of calcium and vitamin D ... *an amount twice or three times* that which nutrition authorities consider essential for preventing deficiency disease. In other words, he says, in addition to a *high calcium diet,* you would do well to supplement it with calcium and vitamin B in other forms—tablets—which may be diminished in four to six months if improvement is satisfactory. The diet may be varied somewhat, but you had better continue giving preference to high calcium foods for the rest of your life, he says. Other high calcium foods are:

Common beans	163 mg.
Beet greens	118 mg.
Chard	105 mg.
Watercress	195 mg.
Dandelion greens	187 mg.
Endive	79 mg.
Kale	225 mg.
Mustard greens	220 mg.
Parsley	193 mg.
Turnip greens	259 mg.

But this is only half the regimen. If you are either developing or already suffering from chronic joint disability, he says there are two other nutritional deficiencies to correct. These are B-complex deficiency and iodine deficiency. Dr. Brady suggests the most potent tablets you can find. He then gives many examples of people helped.

Reported Cases:
- An Ohio woman said she followed the program for about six months. She had been so crippled up with joint disability that she was quite helpless. She declares she is as good as ever now!
- An Ontario woman who gradually got so stiff in all her joints that she couldn't get out of bed or, once she sat up, couldn't lift her feet to finish dressing—adopted the regimen for rheumatism and got relief inside a month. No aches or pains at all now!
- A Minnesota woman says: "You have no idea how my health has improved since I went on the rheumatism regimen. After 4 years in and out of hospitals, loss of work, medications galore, not to mention the suffering I experienced with so-called 'arthritis,' I learned about your regimen. Now I'm feeling my old self again. I don't know what would have become of me. . . ."
- We are told of Mrs. M.A. who had advanced osteoarthritis. She had refused a total hip replacement, and had been living on 60 grains of aspirin daily, for three years. She began taking nine to twelve calcium tablets

daily (about 350 mg. each). Within ten days she was totally free of pain—not one more aspirin!

Garlic Remedies That Have Brought True Miracles!

For centuries, garlic has been hailed as a cure for arthritis. Whether or not this is so, generous amounts of garlic, in the garlic food program—and certain little-known remedies, in which garlic is a prime ingredient—have done wonders in relieving arthritic aches and pains. I do not pretend to know why. It may have something to do with garlic's power to relieve infections, catarrhal swellings and inflammation of the mucous lining of the joints, or its well-known power to increase the circulation, or perhaps some chemical substance or effect not yet discovered. But I do know that garlic remedies for arthritis have worked true miracles.

90% Relief Reported With Garlic!

Aetius, the last renowned physician of the Greco-Roman era, declared that garlic had the power to forestall an attack of gout, particularly in October. Maurice Mességué, in his book *Of Men and Plants*, gives this herbal folklore arthritis remedy, which is not to be eaten:[2]

Garlic (one crushed head)
Greater celandine (leaves, semi-fresh if possible—one handful)
Nettle (leaves and stems, semi-fresh if possible—two handfuls)
Dandelion (whole plant, semi-fresh if possible—one handful)
Meadow sweet (flowers—one handful)
Buttercup (flowers and leaves—one handful)

---

[2]Reprinted with permission of MacMillan Publishing Co., Inc. from *Of Men and Plants* by Maurice Mességué. Copyright © 1972 by Weidenfeld & Nicolson Ltd. Copyright © 1973 by Macmillan Publishing Co., Inc.

Mességué claims 90 percent effectiveness in treating arthritis (30 percent cured, 60 percent greatly improved). This remedy is to be used in the form of foot and hand baths, following the basic instructions on page 37, Chapter 2. He states that while no special diet need be followed, certain foods and drinks (we assume acid-producing sweets and starches, plus coffee and tea) are inadvisable.

Other garlic remedies for arthritis include using it as a tonic or liniment (ordinary vegetable oil in which garlic has been fried is used as a liniment). Reportedly a simple tonic made of diced garlic in a tablespoon of honey, taken with meals over a period of time, can do wonders to relieve pain and suffering, especially in cases of sciatica and gout.

Remedies For Rheumatism and Lumbago!

For myself, my family and friends, garlic has worked true miracles. Some of the soaks and compresses my family and I have used were quite similar to Mességué's, except we substitute garlic for onions, in some cases. The contents are almost identical, and we consider them interchangeable. Onion is milder, and does not enjoy as great a reputation as garlic. Garlic, on the other hand, is often called a "little onion." Here are Mességué's lumbago and rheumatism remedies, which should not be taken internally:[3]

LUMBAGO
Onion (one large grated)
Single-seed hawthorn (blossom—one handful)
Great burdock (flowers and leaves—one handful)
Buttercup (leaves and flowers—one handful)
Nettle (leaves, fresh if possible—one handful)

This, he says, is to be used in compresses over the kidneys (see instructions, page 78) and in foot and hand baths (see instructions, page 37).

---

[3] *Of Men and Plants* by Maurice Mességué, *Op. cit.*

RHEUMATISM
> Onion (one large grated)
> Great burdock (leaves—one handful)
> Spring heath (flowers—one handful)
> Roman camomile (one dozen crushed heads)
> Greater celandine (leaves and stems, semi-fresh if possible—one handful)
> Couch-grass (grated roots—one handful)
> Common broom (flowers—one handful)
> Lavender (flowers—one handful)

Use as follows: make a poultice of cabbage, watercress or kale (see instructions, page 78), coated with a liqueur glass of the preceding preparation. This is to be applied only in the event of an acute attack, to the affected areas, directly to the skin, says Mességué. Otherwise, foot and hand baths are the usual curative treatment, he says. (See instructions, page 37.)

A Universal Panacea?

Of onion, Mességué states: "Certain plants have very complex properties that can either heighten their effect or produce the very opposite; the onion is one such plant. It has a long list of properties—diuretic, stimulant, antiscorbutic, expectorant, antiseptic, resolvent, anti-rheumatic—and is therefore an excellent remedy for constipation, flatulence, chilblains, sores and whitlows. In short, it would seem to be a universal panacea that can be used quite safely.

"But this is not so," he continues. "Relatively recent research has shown that while its high sulfur content makes it effective against rheumatism, it could become harmful in liver cases where there is an allergy to sulfur.[4] The same may be true for garlic. The need for qualified medical advice in all cases is therefore underlined.[5]

---

[4]*Of Men and Plants,* Ibid.
[5]Mességué does not use onion for patients of an excitable or worrying nature, nor for those subject to hemmorrage or shingles. However, no reason is given—and it may be noted that garlic has

Remarkable Results Claimed!

The following three cases, including two sworn statements from doctors—and a sensational cure—are given as testimony to the effectiveness of Mességué's treatment, as reported in his biography, *Of Men and Plants*.[6]

Twenty Years Of Suffering Ended!

In one case, a Dr. Camaret, President of the Menton Medical Association, France, says that his wife was cured of rheumatism, from which she had been suffering for twenty years. Neither the doctor himself nor any of his medical colleagues had been able to bring about any improvement. In other "incurable" cases, says Dr. Camaret, these folk remedies brought about improvement "or cured them completely. These results are undeniable."

"Almost Miraculously Cured Of Rheumatism!"

Another French medical doctor, Dr. Echernier, states: "I certify that as a result of following the course of footbaths prescribed by Mr. Mességué, I was almost miraculously cured of a rheumatic condition which has troubled me for several years and had failed to respond to all other treatments."

Withered Arm Healed!

Mességué describes a patient, Anne-Marie M., 19, who had been born with a short, withered arm that never grew much, was useless, and remained bent back across her chest. She had no feeling in the arm (except during rainy weather,

---

been recommended in many cases of nervous affliction (of which shingles is just one example), and that both garlic and onion were frequently eaten in the past, to cure scurvy, symptoms of which are easy bruising and bleeding (hemorrhaging).

[6]Ibid.

when the bones hurt) and could not move it. She had been to many doctors, none of whom were able to help the paralysis and stunted growth.

This was a new problem for Mességué, who diagnosed the atrophy as a kind of rickets. The most important ingredient in his remedy, he states, was onion ("it's sulfur content makes it very effective against rheumatism"). Other ingredients included wild thyme, stinging nettle, great burdock and parsley—diuretics to eliminate the poisons (onion, too, he says is "a powerful enough diuretic for one to have seen it clear the kidneys of patients with uremia"). Hawthorn and linden blossom were prescribed as mild sedatives. Common camomile was used to calm the nerves. For the atrophy, he used field horsetail in a poultice of cabbage and watercress—which has worked miraculously on animals who could barely stand on their feet. These she was to use in poultices and foot and hand baths.

> **Three months later, she returned miraculously cured! She held out her hand. "Look!" she said, and she picked a sheet of paper off the table with it. "I am so happy!" she cried. "It's so marvellous, I can hardly believe it.... I didn't feel anything the first month.... The second month, I began to feel a tickling sensation ... then little by little ... I could move one finger, then another ..."**

A skeptical witness said, "You mean you couldn't previously move your arm and hand? And now you can?"

"Exactly," she said, and to prove it she pinched him several times. The story appeared in all the Paris newspapers. Anne-Marie's parents said it was like a miracle. Only the doctors who had treated her unsuccessfully refused to believe it. "Nothing can be done," said one. "It is beyond the power of any doctor to correct congenital deformities...."

Other Remedies For Neuralgia and Rheumatism!

An Indian scientist states that the oil extract from garlic, used as a liniment, has always been used with great success in paralytic and rheumatic afflictions. Another doctor states that the pain of rheumatic parts may be much relieved by simply rubbing them with garlic. "It gives excellent results," he says. Another leading scientist and expert on garlic therapy states that, taken internally, garlic quickly calms rheumatic and neuralgic pains.

Possible Effects Of Garlic and Onion On Arthritis!

Now, garlic contains strong substances that may affect each type of arthritis. The sulfur compounds responsible for its strong smell are active against germs. It therefore fights infections, so that its ability to reduce catarrhal swellings and inflammation (as in the mucous lining of joints) may account for its reported effectiveness in relieving rheumatic pain —especially when it is applied right over the area. Garlic is usually rich in potassium, which is so necessary for the contraction of every muscle in the body that a lack of it results in paralysis and constipation. This mineral, along with zinc, manganese, and vitamin B-1, is extremely important in nerve and muscle health, and the carbohydrate metabolism of the body. Pain and muscular stiffness are symptoms of rheumatoid arthritis, fibrositis, and gout (a metabolic ailment).

The *alliin* in garlic attacks streptococcus germs. Almost all cases of rheumatic fever start with a streptococcus infection of the tonsils, nose or throat. By now it should be coming clear why garlic may be so important in these diseases. But we are finished? No, indeed.

Remember gout characterized by an excess of uric acid in the blood? Garlic fights toxic poisons in the body. Even Mességué noted that onion is "a powerful enough diuretic for one to have seen it clear the kidneys of patients with uremia." Garlic is stronger in every respect, so can it be less effective? Uremic poisons don't just appear in the blood from nowhere. They seep into the blood from the intestines, where they arise from germs of putrefaction. Mountains of scientific evidence show that garlic kill germs of putrefaction in the intestines. Is that all? Not by a long shot?

Possible Effect Of Minerals In Garlic On Osteoarthritis

Garlic contains traces of manganese—a mineral needed by humans in microscopic amounts. Manganese is one of four elements (the others are choline, biotin, and a fourth unidentified one) which fights porosis, a deformity of the leg bone, which is characterized by progressive twisting of the bone and slipping of the tendons. A lack of copper, another trace mineral in garlic, may cause ostoeporosis. When copper was given to lab animals in the form of liver, the disorder was completely prevented. A lack of zinc, which is also present in garlic, may lead to bone and joint ailments, studies have shown. All these are present in garlic (salad) foods.

An Octogenarian Kicks Up His Heels!

Mr. J.P. reports: "At the age of 83, I experienced some pain in both knees. I blamed it on the damp weather we were having and on my age. The pain became worse as time went by and there was now a slight swelling on both knees. I ignored it as something unavoidable at my age, and kept as active as I could despite the pain I felt in walking.

"It became torture every morning to bend my knees to put socks on; and sitting for several hours with friends made it so bad I could barely get up and answer the phone, or walk with my friends to the door as they were leaving. They would kid me with, 'old age has finally caught up with you.' As the left knee was the worst, I walked with a slight limp. Then a miracle happened!

"I happened to have some zinc tablets around the house, and rather than waste them I started taking them. To my surprise I noticed a few weeks later that the pain in my knees had become less severe, and the swelling had gone down some. I now began to take one with each meal, and in two months the pain was completely gone as was the swelling.

"We can't go on blaming every ailment that plagues the elderly on old age. Why was I in misery with my knee at the age of 83, but free of the ailment at a few months from 85? Today I can keep stride with my younger friends, kick, jump or run without having any discomfort whatever."

Other Factors In Garlic Foods That May Affect Arthritis!

Garlic foods—the foods with which garlic is normally eaten—such as meats and green, leafy vegetables, are rich in calcium. In September 1953, Dr. L.W. Cromwell of San Diego, California, reported that he had found calcium deficiency to be a cause of arthritic crippling.

Calcium is stored in the bones. In emotional or physical stress, or if you lack calcium, your body draws it from the bones. This may cause osteoporosis, which means brittle bones; or osteomalacia, which is deformed bones. Dr. Cromwell points out that the body compensates for this weakening of the bones by depositing extra calcium at the joints. Excess buildup causes crippling. Adding lots of calcium to the diet, he says, removes the need for thickened joints. The excess is dissolved or reabsorbed—thus easing the condition!

Reportedly, many doctors think that giving calcium to arthritis sufferers will cause more deposits at the joints. Instead, hoping to break up excess deposits, they give cortisone, which is known to carry calcium out of the body. What happens, says one researcher, is that entire bones are weakened, and the body redoubles its efforts to build up the joints. The condition is worsened. One researcher states that giving calcium can relieve the pain of arthritis in one to three days. Calcium helps vitamin C form normal cartilage around joints.

Reported Case:
- Mr. S.P. reports: "My nephew broke his leg over a year ago and has been under the doctor's care, but the break would not heal. Not knowing the exact form of treatment he was getting, I inquired what he was doing. He informed me that he was spending all his mon-

ey for vitamins and drinking a quart of milk per day with no results. I suggested that he take bone meal and if he was not soon walking on his broken leg without crutches, I would pay for the tablets. Three weeks later his mother wrote and told me he had taken the bone meal and had walked a quarter of a mile to her home without his crutches. It is like a miracle."

- In one reported case, a 30-year old woman, Candice C., fell and broke her thigh. It was barely healed enough for her to walk on crutches when it broke again. Expensive surgery was done, and she was given a plastic hip joint. After many months of pain, calcium began to form over the plastic bone! Then she tried an eating plan involving generous amounts of calcium. Within three days, her pain completely disappeared. In a month, she was walking without a limp!

- In another case, John B., 40, fell and broke his thigh. The bones refused to heal. Doctors decided to put in a steel brace. When this was done a bone infection set in. When that refused to heal, an amputation was recommended! None of his doctors had ever told him to eat foots rich in calcium, protein, B vitamins, and vitamin C (what I call garlic foods), but as soon as he did improvement was rapid. He now walks briskly and normally.

A Proven New Home Cure for Arthritis!

As was pointed out previously, strong mental commands can wall out pain to an astonishing degree, some experts going so far as to say that arthritis can be cured by mind power alone! One such expert is Dr. Evelyn Monohan, who says in her book, *The Miracle of Metaphyiscal Healing* (Parker Publishing Co., Inc., 1975) that arthritis, bursitis, and gout can be cured, often immediately, with a technique she gives in detail. Hundreds have been cured, she says!

Her method involves clearly visualizing the cure, in a quiet place, relaxed, eyes closed, visualizing it fading away, with positive affirmations that you are being cured, visualizing doctors and friends congratulating you on that fact, several times a day, completely blotting out all negative thoughts.

Do not be fooled by the simplicity of this method, says Dr. Monohan. It works, when followed faithfully. Even more surprising, she says that this method seems to produce a kind of psychic irradiation that is healing and beneficial to others. In this manner, you can heal others, even at a distance, she says. It is even more powerful if more than one person is concentrating. It never fails, and is 100 percent effective, it used faithfully, she says, and will work just as well for you as it has for others. You can rid yourself of all traces of this disease, she says, offering positive proof that mind power is miracle medicine food for arthritis.

Reported Cases:
- She tells how Susan R., 32, confined to a wheelchair for 2 years due to arthritis of the legs and spine (hopelessly incurable, according to doctors), was given this miracle medicine food and was able to stand up and walk!
- She tells how Katherine T., 50, who had suffered from bursitis in both shoulders for ten agonizing years, was given this miracle medicine food. In three days, the pain disappeared and never returned. X-rays showed no trace of the disease. She was cured! Dr. Monohan gives many other cases cured!

16

Miracle Medicine Foods For New Youth!

Honey has tremendous rejuvenating powers. According to *The Statesman,* one of the leading papers in India, Pandit Madan Mohan Malaviya, 76, went into seclusion one January, and lived on a diet of milk, butter, honey and aonla, resting and meditating for a month and a half.

He was miraculously transformed—from a bent, withered old man, whose face was furrowed with wrinkles, his mouth a gaping toothless cavity—to a robust, younger-looking version of himself, such as friends had not seen in years! His skin was smooth and rosy. New teeth appeared! He looked and felt 20 years younger!

In *Science Digest* for October 1963, there is a two-page photograph of a large group of men, captioned: "Every one of these men is over 100." It says: "In the southern part of the Soviet Union people live a long time. Here is a chorus of 100-year-olds from Abkhazia.... Moreover, these remarkable oldsters are not in the last stages of physical decline, but are as alert and healthy as people from other parts of the world who are 30 or 40 years younger. A Russian team investigating Soviet Georgia reported recently that this relatively small area has 2,000 men aged 100 or more." Many still able to put in a full day's work!

Among these people, it was found that 40 percent of the men over 90 could still see well enough to thread a needle without glasses. Women remained fertile to their sixth decade! And doctors obtained sperm from a man who was 119! "They know no sickness," said one observer. It is reported that favorite foods among these people are *garlic, yogurt, and honey*. One investigator interviewed about 200 of them, inquiring as to their ages, occupations, and diet, and he discovered that most of them were beekeepers. On closer inspection, he discovered that they did not actually eat honey but rather the sediment—or little pieces—which are found at the bottom of a hive, which are deemed unsalable. Analysis reveals that most of this is actually *pollen!* Their staple foods are grains, fruits, raw vegetables, very little milk, eggs or meat, and no refined or processed foods.

The Man Who Lived Two and A Half Centuries!

Professor Li Chung Yun is famous for having lived longer than any other man on record—an incredible 256 years! His death, the cause of which remains unknown, was reported by *The New York Times* in 1933. A professor at Minkuo University claimed to have found records showing Li was born in 1677, and that on his 150th and 200th birthday he was officially congratulated by the Chinese government. He gave a series of 28 lectures on longevity at a Chinese university at the age of 200!

Those who saw him claimed he did not appear older than 52. He stood straight and strong, walked briskly, and had his own hair and teeth! He outlived 23 wives, and was married at the time to his 24th! Early in life, he became interested in herbs. His favorite herbs were ginseng and Fo-Ti-Tieng, taken in the form of teas.

Professor Li advocated a vegetarian diet. His philosophy was "Keep a quiet heart, sit like a tortoise, walk sprightly like a pigeon, and sleep like a dog." Of the herbs he used, ginseng is believed good for the heart, sex glands, stomach, nerves, and blood. Fo-Ti-Tieng's main value (among many valuable properties) seems to be against senility. A Hindu sage named Nanddo Narain, at 107, claimed that Fo-Ti-

Tieng provides a missing ingredient in man's diet which prevents disease and decay. Fo-Ti-Tieng has been called "the Elixir of Life," containing Youth Vitamin X.[1]

Olive Oil and Distilled Water!

Goddard Ezekiel Dodge Diamond, who lived to 120, attributed his long life to olive oil, which he used in food and for external applications for aches and pains, and to the distilled water which he drank. At 40, he had his first bout with illness, an attack of "black measles," the results of which impaired his vision and hearing. After three years, there was still no improvement. He said, "My eyes were very painful, water running from them and a film gathering over them. My hearing was quite dull and growing worse."

At this point, recalling biblical stories, he decided to try pure olive oil. He applied the oil to his eyes and eyelids, and claimed that after two or three applications his vision cleared. So he decided to try it on his ears. "I used the oil freely about the ears externally, and put drops of oil into the ears, holding it there with bits of cotton balls. In a very short time my sight and hearing were entirely restored."

When he reached 60, arthritic stiffness set in. "One day," he said, "I jumped from a wagon to the ground and my joints did not respond with the usual rebound." He tried it again, and "the proof was there, for not only did the knees refuse to rebound, but the backbone cried out in pain." He immediately used his olive oil, in a routine he followed for the rest of his life. Every day, sometimes twice a day, he took a sponge bath with a wet soaped towel, rubbing briskly to stimulate circulation. After rinsing, he applied olive oil to the inside of his joints, under the arms, elbows, knees, insteps and in the groin area. Next he rubbed the oil on his shoulders, spine, hips, knees, bottom of feet, and scalp.

---

[1] Richard Lucas, *Nature's Medicines,* Parker Publishing Co., Inc., 1966.

Past 100, he was doing gymnastics few young men could equal. At 108, he was riding a bicycle and walking 20 miles a day. He attended social events, and on one occasion, at 110, danced most of the evening with a girl of 16![2]

Other Miracle Medicine Foods For Long Life!

It is said that Zora Agha of Turkey lived to the age of 142 on a diet of one meal a day. This meal consisted chiefly of onions and black bread. He toured the U.S. for an American promoter and perished in two years on a diet of hamburgers and french fries.[3]

> One writer reports that in India, he met a holy man who was 187 years old, with evidence to prove it. Two other men, one 102 and the other 110, said they knew him when they were boys. His diet consisted entirely of tropical fruits, including mango.

In another case, a 104-year-old great-great grandmother traveled 72 miles to New York to visit her old neighborhood, without assistance, and claimed that her secret was a teaspoon of crushed garlic and vodka twice daily. "The garlic brings the blood pressure down," she said, "and the vodka helps the circulation."[4] In yet another case, a 90-year-old ice deliverer in New York was still working twelve-hour days, starting at 3 a.m., lugging fifty-pound ice blocks up several flights of stairs. He claimed he ate just one meal a day, around 5 p.m. consisting mostly of a wedge of Italian cheese and a glass of wine. (Yes, he smoked and drank.) These long-lived people have one thing in common; they all seemed to eat very little.

---

[2] Richard Lucas, *The Magic of Herbs in Daily Living*, Parker Publishing Co., Inc., 1972.
[3] Lucas, *Op. Cit.*
[4] Lucas, *Ibid.*

Nearly Dies At 40—Lives To 102!

In the year 1550, Luigi Cornaro wrote his famous *Treatise on Corpulence* in which he recommended moderation in all things, including food. Cornaro was an Italian nobleman, who nearly died before he was 40 because of excessive eating and drinking. He describes his "heavy train of infirmities, including stomach disorders, gout, and almost continual low fever, and a perpetual thirst." He probably had diabetes.

Yet at age 95, he wrote: "I find myself hearty and content, eating with a good appetite and sleeping soundly. All my faculties, at 95, are as good as ever, and in the highest perfection; my understanding is clearer and better than ever, my judgment is sound, my memory is tenacious, and my spirits are good."

He attributes all this to a diet he had been following for many years. At 86, he described it: "The things I eat are: first, bread, panado (a prepared dish containing soaked bread crumbs), some broth with an egg in it, or some other kinds of soup or spoon meat. Of flesh meat, I eat veal, kid and mutton. I eat poultry of every kind. I eat partridges and other birds.... I likewise eat fish... pike and suchlike, amongst fresh water fish." Apparently, it agreed with him (all that he ate totalled 12 ounces daily, including olive oil, and wine). At 70, he says: "One day, while driving at a high rate of speed, I met with an accident. My carriage was overturned, and was dragged quite a distance before the horses could be stopped. Being unable to extricate myself, I was very badly hurt. My head and the rest of my body were painfully bruised, while one of my arms and one of my legs received especially severe injuries. I was brought home, and my family immediately sent for the doctors who... could not help giving their opinion that I would die within three days.... I nevertheless... refused either to be bled or to take any medicine. I merely had my arm and leg straightened, and permitted my body to be rubbed with certain oils.... It followed that, without using any other kind of remedy and without suffering any further ill or change for the worse, I entirely recovered—a thing which... seemed to my doctors nothing less than miraculous."

By the age of 95, Cornaro found that the body needs less and less food, and yet around this time he felt so vigorous he was still able to mount and ride a horse without assistance!

A Case Of Miracle Rejuvenation!

For Grace McB., 64, the change of life was a nightmare. Ugly hair grew on her chin and upper lip. Her lovely auburn hair became streaked with gray. Her skin became dry and furrowed with wrinkles. Crow's feet appeared at her eyes, and the corners of her mouth. She developed ugly jowls and a double chin that flapped hideously, as well as puffy bags under her eyes.

> "I look like a little old man," she sobbed. It was unfortunately true. Her shiny scalp appeared through thinning hairs all over her head. Her hair was receding right over the forehead. A bald patch was developing in back. No amount of fluffing, shaping or combing could hide it. Her once luxuriant hair was not stringy and short, and refused to grow.

For years, she had watched it all happening—with horror. She went the gamut of protein rinses, hair thickeners, estrogen shots, even face-lifting. Nothing helped. Her hair loss increased. She wore wigs, and looked "aged." Now she was even experiencing periods of senile loss of memory. She would repeat herself or forget what she was saying, her keys, names, dates, addresses, things she had to do. When others pointed this out, she felt humiliated and depressed. She would often just sit and stare.

Looks and Feels 20 Years Younger!

After hearing about nature's all-purpose miracle remedy, garlic, she decided to try this miracle rejuvenation plant, in the garlic food program as previously outlined. She had heard how garlic foods are good for hair and skin, and stimulate the hormone glands.

A dramatic change took place. Her complexion improved —became rosy and healthy-looking. Her facial wrinkles, puffiness, jowls and double chin seemed to disappear. Her loose skin became tight and firm as a youngster's. The embarrassing "face fuzz" on chin and lip began to fade away. Her hair began returning to its normal color— became thick, rich and full!

Her quick, sharp memory returned, and she could remember names, dates, and appointments with ease. She became brisk, active and youthful at an age when others are gray and broken! And so can you, say experts! Now you can have abounding vitality, and the abundant vigor and energy that go with it! Now you can cheat time of 20 to 30 years, with nature's own "Youth Elixir."

Miracle Medicine Foods For New Youth!

Many natural foods are what I call garlic foods—foods that go well with garlic. Garlic foods revitalize the skin by cleansing and purifying the bloodstream, relieving it of toxic poisons and "sludge" that can "clog" the river of life. Garlic is itself the greatest cleansing agent of all—and the bulk foods with which it is eaten push intestinal waste material out of the body, break up impacted sludge in the intestines, melt cholesterol deposits in veins and arteries, and help "sweep the body clean"! Blood is the great cellular "lubricant," but it cannot do its job when hindered by years of accumulated waste. Bodies starve!

When circulation is reduced, cut off or made less effective in any way, there is an actual "drying-out" tendency of the cells of the body—like leaves dying on a vine—and

it is this drying out that causes skin to wrinkle, bones to become brittle and hair to lose its softness and color.

Garlic revitalizes the bloodstream—it increases circulation, detoxifies the bloodstream, and brings within itself and other tonic foods (the foods with which it is normally eaten) more of the oxygen, iron, calcium, vitamins, minerals, enzymes and a host of other elements that living tissues need to nourish and revitalize the body. Bodies starve for this life-giving substance called garlic food.

A Revolutionary New Prime-Of-Youth Health Program!

Why let youth slip through your fingers when medical science has proven beyond the shadow of a doubt that you can hold off aging for 10, 20, 30 years or more—and actually reverse the aging process?

> Biologically, there is no reason why you should grow old! Age is not a matter of years. People age and dry up simply because their glands and cells do not get enough liquid refreshment—life-giving oxygen, plasma, lymph and blood nutrients. In most cases they do not get enough simply because their cells are bathing in poisons—wastes are not fully carried out by the blood, so that fresh oxygen and nutrients can be carried in.

Scientifically, there is no reason in the world why you cannot keep your heart, glands, digestion and all vital organs in perfect working order, and live a hearty, vigorous life filled to the brim with strength, joy and radiant good health until you are well over 100, if the body is fed well and completely cleansed of all impurities. Poisons in the system are the only reason for degeneration of any kind.

Dr. Alexis Carrell proved this way back in 1911 by keeping the cells of a chicken heart alive for 30 years! He did this by placing them in a solution containing everything needed for life, and thoroughly cleansing them every 48 hours! His associates continued the experiment, and the heart muscles are still alive and beating to this day!

You'll See and Feel The Results Almost Overnight!

Perhaps you cannot cleanse your body of every poison (although I really believe that nothing is incurable), but you *can* drastically reduce the effect of years of accumulated waste from junk food and poor living habits with the garlic food program—surround every tiny cell with all the life-giving elements it needs and add perhaps up to 30 health-packed years to your life, starting now!

Garlic has a "tonic" effect on every area of the body—from skin surfaces to the tissues, cells and vessels deep inside—and when you eat garlic and garlic foods, you experience what doctors call the "tonic response"—a sense of invigoration—a state of mind and body so spectacular that it actually helps you fight off the disease of middle and old age!

Nature will amaze you as she restores your body in a fraction of the time it took to get that way in the first place. You will feel decades younger, and this can happen almost overnight. You'll see the results, you'll feel the results, your friends will applaud the results, in the first ten days alone. You'll discover a new "you" you never thought existed—because when you feel great and look great the world is your oyster!

Circles Under The Eyes Vanish!

Even in advanced age you can be healthy and your appearance can fool the calendar. Often, with the garlic food program, you can actually feel the years roll back as every tiny cell in your body fills out and grows young and firm again. Headaches, tired blood, leg congestion, varicose veins and impotence caused by blood-starved sex cells, can become a thing of the past, as I have shown in previous chapters! Take the case of Gerold O., nearing seventy!

> Gerold O.'s skin hung in loose folds. His chin sagged and he suffered from blemishes and dark circles under his eyes that made him look old and haggard. With the garlic food program, his skin speedily firmed up. Blemishes subsided. His loose skin became tight. His "sagging chin" was firm as a youngster's!

How can this happen? The answer is simple and obvious. Dark circles under the eyes are caused by bluish oxygen-starved blood, which can actually be seen through the thin skin below the eyes. (There is no layer of fat beneath the skin surrounding the eyes—it is very thin and almost transparent, and highly flexible to permit quick eye movement.) The blood flowing under it can be seen and it is blue rather than red when the blood lacks oxygen and accumulates carbon dioxide, a poisonous waste.

This results from many conditions which garlic foods can relieve. Lack of sleep, tiredness, fatigue or nervous exhaustion can cause it. Garlic is an excellent sleeping potion and nerve tonic. Excess germs of putrefaction in the intestines may cause it. Garlic is the greatest germ-fighter. Incorrect eating habits may cause it. Foods which raise the carbon dioxide content of the blood include cakes, pies, pastries, pudding, ice cream, bread, candy, and alcoholic beverages (anything with too much sugar or starch, the carbohydrate foods, will reportedly darken the blood, causing dark circles or blue shadows under the eyes). But plenty of garlic foods, including fresh fruits and vegetables, will reportedly make the blood redder, causing these eye shadows to fade away.

In addition, garlic foods soothe the liver—which always brightens the complexion—help make fatty deposits melt away, and have a "tonic," tightening or bracing effect on loose, flabby skin. As the skin firms up, wrinkles and creases fade away. Garlic is diuretic (i.e., it gently stimulates sluggish kidneys), and the high potassium content of garlic and the foods with which it is eaten help the body excrete excess fluids. Therefore, bloating, puffiness, bags under the eyes tend to diminish. Convinced?

A Power Source Of Natural and Instant Health!

The garlic food program is the normal way, the safe way, the natural and inexpensive way to get the cellular lubrication you need. It is a step-by-step, look-younger, feel-better, live-longer program based on scientific fact, medical endorsement, and a staggering array of successes!

The beauty of garlic is that within minutes after you eat this substance, it is speeding to work in cells, tissues and organs! The same may be said of garlic foods (the foods with which it is eaten). They, too, are speedily digested, assimilated, and absorbed to nourish and regenerate your body!

It is a power source of natural and instant health. The cleansing and nutrition secret, which Dr. Carrel discovered —and which garlic foods accomplish so well—is one that doctors have been whispering the praises of for years! It is the secret of youthful looks and vigorous long life that millions the world over have been clamoring to learn about. They pursue this goal every day in expensive European health spas and beauty salons—without any hope of ever achieving it because they do not know this secret. Garlic foods are not a fad. They have been around a long time. Unlike some so-called "wonderdrugs" that are rushed onto the market without adequate testing, garlic is inexpensive and effective, proven safe a thousand times over. "Let food be your medicine and medicine your food"—as long as it is garlic food, we might add.

Youth Restorative "X": A Cure For Aging!

What is the "mysterious" youth secret of garlic that has caused it to be hailed as a cure for aging in every civilization since the dawn of time? More than any secret youth substance it contains—and it contains several—I believe it is a secret ingredient which all miracle medicine foods have, and which I call Youth Restorative "X".

Miracle Youth Restorative "X" is the natural cleaning power of all "living" foods, in contrast to "dead" chemically processed foods. In this case it is garlic's triple threat as an antibiotic, anti-aging, anti-senility youth restorative due mainly, I believe, to the combined forces of garlic and vitamin B-1, which combine to form allithiamin.

It is this scientifically proven power, along with its high potassium content, and all the other vitamins, minerals, enzymes, catalysts, and nutrients in garlic and garlic foods, that account for garlic's reputation as a miracle youth resorative.

The Anti-Senility Food!

I keep coming back to garlic's thiamin-boosting power, simply because this relatively recent (1961) discovery helps to explain so much about garlic's reputed powers. Take memory and learning, for example.

If garlic increases your absorption of vitamin B-1 (thiamin)—and it does—that would mean that garlic has an antisenility factor. How do we know that garlic, by way of vitamin B-1, can clear the mind? In 1938, Bruno Minz, working at the laboratory of the Sorbonne University in Paris, discovered that a cut nerve ending exudes a liquid that contains thiamin. He further found that when a nerve is electrically stimulated, it gives off 80 times as much thiamin.

Years later, Dr. Ruth Flinn Harrell, at Johns Hopkins Hospital, discovered that when brain-damaged patients received added vitamin B-1 in their diet, they recovered much more rapidly. In her experiments, she discovered that by giving thiamin to a group of patients, in one month:

- **Memory improved 25%**
- **Hearing improved 25%**
- **Intelligence improved 25%**

With that in mind, garlic's ability to increase the body's absorption of vitamin B-1 *ten times as much* (an amount otherwise impossible except by liquid injections) takes on great importance. In so doing, it may also increase your absorption of other B vitamins.

A Diet For Youthfulness!

Vitamin B-1, if taken apart from the other B complex vitamins in increased amounts, can cause induced deficiencies in the rest. Vitamin B-1 is most readily available—with all the others—in high B complex foods such as brewer's yeast and garlic foods—lean pork, liver and kidneys (the organ meats) and lima beans (foods that go well with garlic). In fact, many B-vitamins present in these foods, such as pyridoxine (B-6), DNA, RNA, folic acid and pantothenic acid, are often missing from B complex pills of the drug store type. In 1972, interesting work was reported along these lines.

> **Benjamin Frank, M.D., a leading researcher, used a complete dietary program of vitamin B-rich foods to slow down, halt, and even reverse the aging process. Brewer's yeast, which he says is rich in nucleic acid, is the cornerstone of this program—which includes desiccated liver, large quantities of sardines, sweetbreads, and supplementary B vitamins and minerals. This was tested on people ranging in age from 40 to 70!**

If the reported results are any indication, think how much more effective this method would be with garlic—and its power to speed absorption of B-1 tenfold—added. Immediate results included an increase in energy and well-being, especially with high doses. Rapid effects were noted within 48 hours.

Wrinkles Diminished, Skin Smoother!

The most striking effect was on the skin of the face. Within a week the skin became smooth, soft, and young-looking, with a rosy glow. Within a month or so, wrinkles, lines and age spots began to fade away. Other areas began to show improvement. Roughened elbows became smoother, hands became younger looking.

Heart and Memory Improved!

Other organs besides the skin were affected. In older patients with coronary heart disease and congestive heart failure, the heart function was clearly improved. Significant effects were noted with regard to the brain, which responded with an increase in mental alertness and improved memory.

A Cure For Senility?

M.L. Mitra, medical assistant at Nether Edge and Winter Street Hospitals in Sheffield, England, believes that much of what passes for "senility" is simply a lack of B and C vitamins in the diet. To illustrate his point, he presents 28 case histories of patients admitted to a hospital "old age" ward in a confused state (*Journal of the American Geriatrics Society*, June 1971). After treatment, 21 were sent home completely normal.

> He found that all the patients had one thing in common: a vitamin deficiency. Many were 80 years old, or older, and had been living alone. For most, fixing a balanced meal was just "too much trouble." Seventeen were suffering from thiamin/vitamin B complex deficiencies; two others had pellagra (a niacin deficiency). Seven had low vitamin C. Many were living on a diet consisting entirely of potatoes and a few slices of bread and jam.

Massive doses of B-complex and C vitamins were given by mouth and by injection. In case after case, spectacular cures were reported!

Reported Cases:
- F.B., an 88-year-old female, lived alone and ran her own lodging home. She was admitted to the hospital because of severe dehydration and a confused mental

state. She had been taking a drug, chlorpromazine, for the mental condition, but she was still confused. She was given a concentrated dose of B complex vitamins. Her confusion disappeared, she regained her mental faculties, and was able to return home.
- R.M., a 76-year-old female, also lived alone. Admitted to the hospital with an eye ailment—paralysis of the eye muscles—she suddenly became very confused. Her doctor made a long, complicated diagnosis, indicating brain disease. Mitra simply gave her B complex vitamins, and her mental state improved so dramatically that she was discharged in two weeks.
- R.C., a 95-year-old female, lived with her bachelor son who was away from home a lot. She had been treated with diuretics for congestive heart failure. She was admitted to the hospital in a confused mental state, complaining of intense bone tenderness and many bruises (symptoms of vitamin C deficiency). After treatment with a gram of vitamin C daily for two weeks, she improved so much she was discharged home.
- A.P., an 83-year-old woman, was admitted to the hospital in a confused mental state. She was found to be suffering from bronchial pneumonia, but remained confused even after recovery. "However, the confusion cleared completely after treatment with vitamin B complex orally," Mitra writes.

Many such studies have been conducted on the effect of B and C vitamins in combatting senility. The findings are all similar. But many—perhaps most—doctors refuse to accept these findings without years of further study, exploring every possible angle. They can't even agree as to what constitutes senility. Whatever the definition—confusion, loss of memory, a tendency to repeat oneself—early signs of mental deterioration seem to clear up with vitamin therapy, say other experts.

Diet Change Cured Psoriasis, Darkened Hair, Improved Eyes!

Mr. N.D. writes: "About 2 years ago, I had the misfortune to develop one of the worst cases of sore hands that

I have ever seen. The skin on my hands turned a dark red color and they were so dry that the slightest pressure caused the skin to crack open. The condition was limited to the palms at this time. I sought help from a dermatologist and the diagnosis was a form of psoriasis. I was given a prescription for cortisone ointment to be applied each night, and told to wear plastic and cotton gloves while sleeping. I followed this advice for three months, at the end of which time the condition was spreading to my fingers and wrists.

"I then came to the conclusion that my problem was probably caused by a very strict diet which I had been advised to follow to control a high cholesterol count. I decided to give up the prescribed treatment and started eating some eggs and fats and oils. I also started taking vitamin supplements every day, including vitamin E, B complex, cod liver oil capsules, and vitamin C with bioflavonoids.

"At the end of three months my hands were completely cured. In addition, I received unexpected bonuses. My gray hair is beginning to darken and I passed my eye examination for a driver's license without my glasses. Needless to say, I am continuing my new diet and taking natural vitamins."

Massage Is Miracle Medicine
Food That Restored Hair!

R.N. reports: "Two years ago I decided to do something about my thinning hair. For years it kept getting thinner and thinner. I had a receding part going back an inch or more and all my hair was getting thin on top (I'm 55). I tried wigs, but I couldn't stand them.

"I decided to massage my scalp for one minute every morning without using any gooky preparation. One minute doesn't seem long, but when you watch a clock to make sure of the time, your arms can get pretty tired. But I kept on, and even if I forgot on weekends, I did it every day as part of my daily work.

"To my surprise I noticed all new hair coming in around my receding part, about a quarter to an half inch long. This was about three months after I began massaging. At this time I feel my hair is thicker and the indentation I had at the part in my hair has filled in to the normal line."

How To Stop Falling Hair
(Another Form Of Massage)

Nerve massage can be miracle medicine food for your hair, one expert claiming that it will not only stop your falling hair, but will help you grow a new head of hair, even if you are now bald! It consists of rubbing the fingernails of one hand directly across the fingernails of the other, briskly, for five minutes three times a day. In a few weeks, says this expert, hair loss will cease, and you'll have plenty of hair, and never a gray hair, as long as you live. Thousands of people 60 and 70 years of age, are living proof that it works, says this expert!

One man who claimed that baldness ran in his family, used this miracle medicine food for the hair (nerve massage) and says: "Soon my head began to have a fuzz, and then the hair began to grow, and now at over 70 years of age I have a fine luxurious head of hair."

Garlic Grows New Hair!

Garlic has been employed for centuries as an effective remedy for baldness or bald spots. Here are two methods of application, which can reportedly work wonders in stimulating new hair growth.

1. Slice open a clove of garlic lengthwise, and rub on the affected area, squeezing out the juice. Allow to dry. Mix a few drops of bay rum and olive oil and massage with this an hour later. Apply once in the morning and again at night.
2. Dice two cloves of garlic very finely and mash well. Mix into a pint of 90 proof alcohol. Allow to stand for two days. Strain. Add one cup of fresh burdock,

chopped roots or flower heads. Allow to stand for five days. Strain. Sponge onto scalp every evening for a month. Reportedly, this is sufficient to promote hair growth.

The story is told of two men, both nearing 75, who used a much simpler—though somewhat antisocial—method of employing garlic's hair-growing properties. They simply rubbed in the juice of a thin slice of garlic on the affected areas and allowed it to dry. This was done three times a day. In a few weeks, reportedly, the bald or balding patches were all filled in with an "abundant crop of hair"!

Possible Effects Of Garlic On Hair!

Naturally, the hair roots must still be alive, but my theory is that the reason it worked is twofold. First, as many doctors have acknowledged, garlic is a well-known rubefacient (capable of stimulating blood circulation—and also containing all the nutrients that hair follicles need), with strong penetrative powers. Secondly, the mineral content may have had something to do with it. Garlic is rich in sulfur—which accounts for its smell—and human hair contains lots of sulfur. Garlic also has zinc; when experimental animals are deprived of zinc in the diet, they invariably go bald. It contains copper. The graying of hair has been produced experimentally by a lack of copper. Finally, garlic increases your absorption of B vitamins when you eat foods that go well with it, and B vitamins have been found to cause hair to darken, in actual lab tests on scientists themselves.

Two Hair-Raising Experiences!

The experience of Mrs. K.L. seems to bear out my theory. She tells of a method of feeding which grew fur on three bald spots on a little four-year-old dog: "The runt of the litter, he had had plentiful (black) fur except that a big spot on his back, the top of his head, and his ears were bald. He also had severe sinus drainage. I had been reading about zinc, and decided to see what supplemental feeding would do. Each day he was given four half-inch hamburger balls into which had been inserted a clove of garlic, quartered, a brewer's yeast tablet (rich in B vitamins), zinc with kelp, a bone meal tablet and a vitamin C tablet, plus his other food. At the end of two months he very rarely had sinus drainage, he was a bouncy little dog with no nervous shaking fits, and had velvety black fur on all bald areas, with white hairs filling in the outer edge of all bald spots."

"Several years ago," said Lawrence O., "I noticed that my hair was receding right over the forehead—in an embarrassing 'V'—and around the sides, the hair near my temples was almost all gone. Several people had pointed out a bald spot that I was developing right in the back of my head. The rest of my hair was quite gray. I was embarrassed, frightened and humiliated. I didn't want to look old before my time.

"Then I remembered an old-world remedy using garlic. I simply rubbed it on the affected areas every night. After a few weeks, my forehead and temples were filling in! By summer, the bald patch had grown in again! It was a miracle. And I noticed dark roots all over. I looked and felt years younger."

This case is unverified but reportedly true, and was told to me many years ago by a man in his *seventies*, with thick wavy black hair, who looked no more than 50 or 55. He said he'd never lost a day of work, never felt better since he started eating only natural foods at age 50, and did not plan to retire.

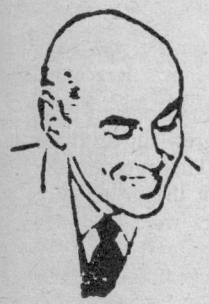 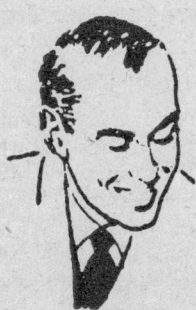 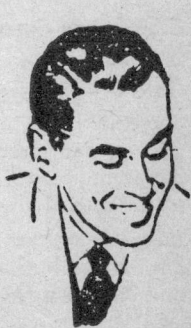

Impossible? While doctors violently object that male-pattern baldness is completely incurable—there are astounding reports of new hair growth with power-packed Miracle Medicine Foods!

One researcher reports many cases where Miracle Medicine Foods caused new hair to grow again even in advanced cases of baldness. A typical case is Ty H., a middle-aged man, bald for 20 years. No scalp disease or illness, just bald. The baldness extended deep back, with just a gray fringe around the edges, and looked completely hopeless. He began eating only natural, unprocessed foods, with the result that in two weeks, dark hair started coming in! In a little over a month, most of the back and top had started filling in!

In a major breakthrough, male-pattern baldness has been almost 100 percent cured or stopped in cases tested with vitamin B-6 (biotin) and amino acids. The vitamin B-6 helps dissolve excess testosterone—the male hormone—on the scalp, and combines with amino acids to build up the hair roots.

Spectacular cures have been reported. Men losing nearly 500 hairs a day had fallout reduced to as little as 25 (45 a day is normal). One man reports his hairline restored as much as two inches in the front. All this happened in a matter of weeks!

Thousands Experience New Hair Growth!

In another case, a man we'll call Martin D. was completely bald on top except for a few long hairs. It seemed incredible to him that the thick wavy hair in his high school picture had disappeared in just a few short years. It started innocently enough, with a little extra hair in his comb every day. He tried massaging his scalp to improve the circulation.

His hair continued to fall out. Nearly 30, he could see and feel the thinning process, as each day his hairline

receded more. Huge wads appeared in his [obscured] could pull them out with his fingers. Sometimes [obscured] just fell out and landed on his shirt. People began to notice. He frantically tried heat lamps, oil treatments and ointments—you name it, he tried it!

He tried to relax to relieve scalp tension. He heard conflicting reports that too much washing caused dryness, or that too little caused excess oil to clog the hair roots, cutting off life and growth. He read that soap with too much lye caused damage, and switched to milder shampoos, rinsing thoroughly. He made a real effort to keep his hands off his hair—and to avoid excess combing. He thought of decreasing sexual activity, on the theory that he was losing vital hormones and minerals, or having more sex, to reduce excess male hormones —leaving more female hair-growing hormones in his body. All failed. By the time he was past 50, he was completely bald.

Miraculous New Hair Growth!

Then he began reading about nutrition. He began taking vitamins and minerals, including 24,000 units of vitamin A from fish liver oils, once a day, and the following three times daily: one kelp tablet, four high-potency B complex tablets, 100 units of vitamin E complex, two tablets of iron and liver concentrate, two multivitamin and mineral tablets. If this seems a lot, remember that he had a history of sluggish glands and many health problems. He decided to eliminate all junk foods.

The once-shiny pate developed downy fuzz that seemed to thicken and grow darker each day. Hairs sprang forth that he hadn't seen in years. The crown above his forehead and in his back began filling in. In just a few weeks he noticed dark hair at the temples.

A typical breakfast included two eggs (soft, poached or scrambled), a slice of protein bread with soya lecithin spread, raw wheat germ and sunflower seed meal mixed with half a season. He began eating lean meats, fish ...getables, green salads, cottage cheese, a tea-...ay—totalling three—of wheat germ oil, soya, ...r other vegetable oils, and carrot juice whenever ... His diet included beef, liver, organ meats, baked ... potatoes, apricots, fresh unsalted nuts, cucumbers—in o..er words, the garlic food program (foods that go well with garlic).

Over a period of 18 months, the hair lengthened and thickened, making it possible for him to comb it. At this time, he was doing so well that he was able to reduce some of his supplements like B complex, vegetable and wheat germ oil by half or less, and could eat less meat. During the next 18 months, it was obvious that a completely new crop of hair was coming in. It made him look and feel years younger. And we are told that younger men with fewer health problems have accomplished the same thing practically overnight, or in a matter of weeks!

Many Claim Hair Darkens!

William Brady, M.D. was a syndicated writer whose health columns were read by millions. In his book, *An Eighty Year Old Doctor's Secrets of Positive Health* (Prentice-Hall, 1961), he recommends iodine food supplements for the many symptoms of iodine deficiency. However, people who read his column and tried it reported that the most startling effect was a darkening of the hair. In their letters they refer to a commercial brand called *Neoco Iodin Ration, Improved,* which was apparently an iodine tablet available in the California area. For them it was Miracle Medicine Food!

Reported Cases:
- "I had never seen gray hair get back its natural color, but mine did after using the Iodin Ration. I believe our soil (French West Africa) lacks iodine..."—C.A.
- "We live in the Great Lakes region and are users of the Iodin Ration. My hair was a startling white but now it's doing its darndest to be black again, its original color."—J.W.

- "Taking the Iodin Ration two years. My hair, which used to be brown, has turned nearly black. Always had wavy hair but now it is curly, so curly that friends think I have a permanent."—Mrs. K.R.
- "Your Iodin Ration has been included in my daily diet for about a year and never before have I had such nice hair, and it's so manageable. I am 58 and the gray hairs I have had disappeared."—Mrs. B.A.
- "My hair has been restored to original color in the two years I have been on Iodin Ration. I can find no explanation for this except the Iodin Ration."—Mrs. H.W.
- "Foolishly I let my Iodin Ration run out and within two months my hair became dry and dull, several white hairs appeared ... now I'm back on Iodin Ration; hair has regained its dark color and is shining again. I am most grateful..."—J.S.F.
- "My daughter, 24, had always had straight stringy hair. Last summer her hair, on top, was taking on a natural wave and by Thanksgiving the sides as well were beginning to curl. Now it has a lovely wave of its own, without the aid of curlers...."—Mrs. W.M.

If miracle medicine foods can grow new hair, and darken white hair, can they also do all the astonishing things in this book? "YES!" says thousands of users!

Another Case Of Miracle Rejuvenation!

Mr. G.E. reports: "About three years ago, at 64 years of age, my hair was snow-white. I was becoming crippled with arthritis in both shoulders and my right hand. Then I had a heart attack. The doctor said quit work, retire, and take it easy if I wanted to live. But I had to earn a living. Then, a short time later, the final blow came: a serious and extremely painful jawbone infection. The dentist said that because of my heart condition, they didn't dare do anything for me, so I wound up in the hospital as an emergency case. This forced me to retire. For about a year and a half, I was virtually helpless.

"A few minutes of work or exertion of any kind, and I would be deathly sick that evening. So I started reading books on health foods, vitamin and mineral supplements. Shortly afterwards, I threw away the medicines prescribed by the doctor. These chemicals had not effected any cure, and some side effects were bad.

"The results, after two years of the proper foods, plus vitamin and mineral supplements in much larger amounts than the minimum recommended, are: the once snow-white hair is rapidly turning black again. I seldom have any arthritic twinges any longer. I no longer have any sign of heart trouble. My strength is virtually back to where it was 20 years ago, and in some ways better than it was 20 years ago. I now go swimming, usually a couple of times a week, and enjoy a healthy vigorous life."

Need I say more? All over America, miracles are happening with Miracle Medicine Foods! Described here are tough, resistant, hard-to-heal conditions deemed incurable by doctors—cases where all else failed—that were completely and permanently cured, or apparently abated, with no sign of return. No cancer cure is claimed, and self-medication is not recommended, but if your doctor approves, what has worked for others may work for you.

And, of course, remember garlic, the Miracle Medicine Food that is remarkably similar to penicillin. Unlike penicillin, available only in doctor-prescribed drugs that may cause serious side-effects or allergic reaction—this plan is safe and available without prescription, and can be eaten for enjoyment.

Bon appetit!

Improve Your Health with Warner Books

__LOW SALT SECRETS FOR YOUR DIET
by Dr. William J. Vaughan   (L37-223, $3.95, U.S.A.)
(L37-358, $4.50, Canada)

Not just for people who must restrict salt intake, but for everyone! Forty to sixty million Americans have high blood pressure, and nearly one million Americans die of heart disease every year. Hypertension, often called the silent killer, can be controlled by restricting your intake of salt. This handy pocket-size guide can tell you at a glance how much salt is hidden in more than 2,600 brand-name and natural foods.

__EARL MINDELL'S VITAMIN BIBLE
by Earl Mindell   (L30-626, $3.95, U.S.A.)
(L32-002, $4.95, Canada)

Earl Mindell, a certified nutritionist and practicing pharmacist for over fifteen years, heads his own national company specializing in vitamins. His VITAMIN BIBLE is the most comprehensive and complete book about vitamins and nutrient supplements ever written. This important book reveals how vitamin needs vary for each of us and how to determine yours; how to substitute natural substances for tranquilizers, sleeping pills, and other drugs; how the right vitamins can help your heart, retard aging, and improve your sex life.

__SUGAR BLUES
by William Dufty   (30-512, $3.95)

Like opium, morphine, and heroin, sugar is an addictive drug, yet Americans consume it daily in every thing from cigarettes to bread. If you are overweight, or suffer from migraine, hypoglycemia or acne, the plague of the Sugar Blues has hit you. In fact, by accepted diagnostic standards, *our entire society is pre-diabetic. Sugar Blues* shows you how to live better without it and includes the recipes for delicious dishes—all sugar free!

For Every Kitchen

___THE ALLERGY COOKBOOK & FOOD-BUYING GUIDE
Pamela P. Nonken and   *(L37-901, $7.95, U.S.A.)*
S. Roger Hirsch, M.D.   *(L37-902, $9.95, Canada)*

Pamela Nonken, whose daughter is allergic to yeast, determined to devise a workable diet that included bread products but excluded yeast... and one so delicious that all her family could enjoy it too. She succeeded so well that Dr. Roger Hirsch, a practicing allergist, asked her to expand her efforts and design recipes that would exclude five other common allergens—corn, soy, wheat, eggs, and milk.

___THE CAROB WAY TO HEALTH   *(L37-302, $5.95, U.S.A.)*
Frances Sheridan Goulart   *(L37-315, $7.25, Canada)*

If chocolate doesn't like you, try Mother Nature's perfect treat: carob, the chocolate taste-alike that's everything you ever dreamed about—and less. It's all here, from the wonderpod's ancient history to its uses in cooking and herbal medicine—dozens of delectable recipes for main dishes and accompaniments, frostings, fillings, sauces, beverages, and, of course, candies and snacks.

___THE GOOD HEART DIET COOKBOOK
Ellen Stern & Jonathan Michaels   *(L37-547, $6.95, U.S.A.)*
Foreword by Siegfried J. Kra, M.D.   *(L37-212, $8.50, Canada)*

Who needs this book? All of you who... can't sit through a movie without buttered popcorn, like your asparagus with hollandaise, grab a burger and a soda for a quick bite, have hypertension, are diabetic, have a high cholesterol count, have a family history of heart disease, have arthritis, or are overweight.

HELPFUL READING
FROM WARNER BOOKS

THE EYE/BODY CONNECTION *(L37-599, $9.95, U.S.A.)*
by Jessica Maxwell *(L37-600, $10.95, Canada)*
Your eyes forecast the onset of disease—and your eyes reveal the effects of stress, diet, and heredity on your body. This book presents 59 eye photographs and their readings that will tell you what to look for in your own eyes. The charts enable you to pinpoint vital areas by matching flaws in your iris with points on the diagrams. This is the first book on this subject for laymen and will provide you with a valuable diagnostic tool to the earliest signs of physical disorder.

YOUR BODY DOESN'T LIE *(L30-859, $3.50, U.S.A.)*
by Dr. John Diamond *(L30-873, $4.50, Canada)*
Ask your body what's best for your health. The new science of Behavioral Kinesiology gives you a simple muscle test that discloses your body's individual response to stress, posture, food, emotion, and your social and physical environment. Dr. Diamond shows how the Thymus Gland regulates body energy and can guide you to a healthier way of life.

HOW TO STOP SMOKING IN THREE DAYS
by Sidney Petrie with
Florence Rhyn Serlin, Ph.D. *(30-496, $2.50)*
HOW TO STOP SMOKING IN THREE DAYS is written by two outstanding authorities in the field of hypnosis with extensive practical experience in its use to prevent smoking. Let the secrets of self-hypnosis work for you! You can break the cigarette habit in just 72 hours. Now discover how to use your own best friend—yourself—to open the way to a healthier, longer life!

FUN from
WARNER BOOKS

__ **DC SUPER HEROES SUPER HEALTHY COOKBOOK**
by Mark Saltzman, *Available in hardcover:*
Judy Garlan, & Michelle Grodner *(L51-227, $8.95)*
The most terrific cookbook ever—delicious, easy-to-make, nutritious food presented by all your favorite superheroes. A delight in full-color and in a permanent binding, you will discover how to make everything from breakfast and snacks, to main meals and parties.

__ **RICHARD SIMMONS'**
NEVER-SAY DIET COOKBOOK *(L37-078, $7.95, U.S.A.)*
by Richard Simmons *(L37-553, $9.50, Canada)*
Phase two of Simmons' fat-fighting world plan! This companion volume to his first book presents a comprehensive program for enjoying life's culinary pleasures while staying healthy and shedding excess pounds.

To order, use the coupon below. If you prefer to use your own stationery, please include complete title as well as book number and price. Allow 4 weeks for delivery.

WARNER BOOKS
P.O. Box 690
New York, N.Y. 10019

Please send me the books I have checked. I enclose a check or money order (not cash), plus 50¢ per order and 50¢ per copy to cover postage and handling.*

_____ Please send me your free mail order catalog. (If ordering only the catalog, include a large self-addressed, stamped envelope.)

Name _____

Address _____

City _____

State _____ Zip _____

*N Y State and California residents add applicable sales tax.